RIDING
BARRANCA

RIDING BARRANCA

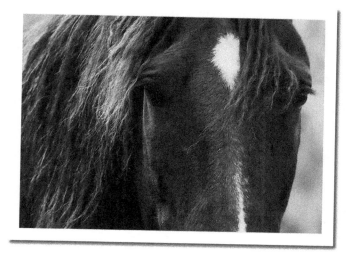

Finding freedom and forgiveness on the midlife trail

Laura Chester

With photographs by **Donna DeMari** & **Mason Rose**

TRAFALGAR SQUARE
North Pomfret, Vermont

First published in 2013 by
Trafalgar Square Books
North Pomfret, Vermont 05053

Disclaimer of Liability
The author and publisher shall have neither liability nor responsibility to any person or entity with respect to any loss or damage caused or alleged to be caused directly or indirectly by the information contained in this book. While the book is as accurate as the author can make it, there may be errors, omissions, and inaccuracies.

Trafalgar Square Books encourages the use of approved safety helmets in all equestrian sports and activities.

Library of Congress Cataloging-in-Publication Data

Chester, Laura.
Riding Barranca : finding freedom and forgiveness on the midlife trail / Laura Chester.
pages cm
ISBN 978-1-57076-578-0
1. Horsemanship—Psychological aspects. 2. Human-animal relationships. 3. Nature, Healing power of. I. Title.
SF309.C468 2013
615.8'51581--dc23 2012049869

Book design by Michelle Thompson | Fold & Gather Design
Cover design by RM Didier
Typefaces: Fiesole, Florence

Printed in the United States of America

10 9 8 7 6 5 4 3 2 1

*to the memory
of my mother, Margaret Sheftall Chester
at long last*

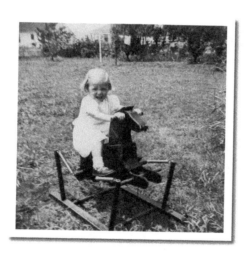

CONTENTS

FOREWORD

by Thomas Moore

I don't know why I am so enchanted by this book by Laura Chester. I'm not a horse person, though after reading the book, I wish I were. If it were a simple book about horses or about various rides taken during the course of a year, I could treat it lightly and let it go. But it is much more than a chronicle or diary. Laura punctuates the rides with unsettling stories of her family, especially her father and mother, and the stories are not all nice. She doesn't tell us how or why her father was a renegade husband. But she's clear that her mother was a difficult person. The counterpoint of horses and family makes this book unusually satisfying. This intrigue, the unanswered questions, the mysterious juxtapositions, are what make this book, to me, a work of art.

I've known Laura for over twenty-five years. Though we haven't seen each other much in a long while, I feel that we've never lost a sense of being colleagues, not only as writers but as pilgrims on this odd path of life. Maybe this connection with her accounts in part for the pleasure I felt in reading her words. It helps that she's a very good writer.

I've often wondered what an animal is. We assume all kinds of things, but I've never felt satisfied with any philosophy of animals. They are like us in many ways. They have some talents that place them above us, especially the power of their senses, and some that seem to place them below us, especially their lack of speech. But when you live with animals, as I have done for fourteen years now with our dog, you know that they have emotions and some kind of thoughts. They can relate and inspire love. You can argue with them and also worry about their safety. I appreciate the places in this book where Laura tells us what a horse is experiencing. I trust her on this.

Recently I read from one of my favorite Zen masters, Shunryu Suzuki, that he'd like to be a frog, able to sit perfectly still for a long time, and when a fly zips by, gulp it down. He doesn't want to eat flies, but he'd like the capacity for sitting and the quick alertness. I think I might like to be a horse, at least the kind that Laura describes, and especially if I had a rider like her.

There's something mysterious about the joining of human and horse. Old stories tell of horsemen arriving at a community where people had never seen horses before. At first, rider and horse looked like one being, a centaur. That's an intimate bond. To me, a psychotherapist, it means a lot to know that for the Greeks one of the prime educators, especially in the field of medicine, was the Centaur Chiron.

Maybe today when a person rides a horse, she becomes a centaur. There were female centaurs in myth. Maybe it's the blend of human and horse that unleashes the healing power. I get that sense in this book, especially toward the end, when there is an unexpected and beautiful passage of forgiveness. I wonder if this was the purpose of the book, conscious or unconscious, to find family healing through companionship with horses. As in myth, the centaur heals—woman and horse.

Thomas Moore
Author of *Care of the Soul*;
Soul Mates; *A Religion of One's Own*

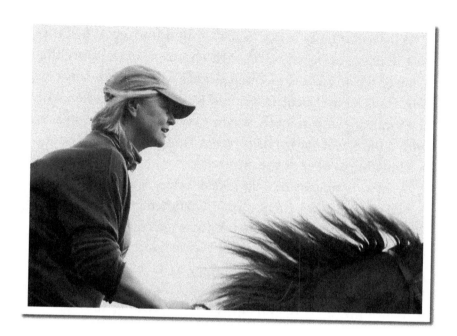

PREFACE

Unconfined space and a feeling of freedom are what I love most about riding. Sinking into the rhythm of the horse, I am more in touch with my instinctive self—more alert to my surroundings, much like the forgiving animal beneath me. I enjoy exploring new territory, not sure of what challenge might face me next. Even getting lost in the wilderness has its own rewards—reminding me that I am never completely in charge—that the earth is a huge, magnificent place full of surprises. More often than not, I have found that my horse has a better sense of direction than I do. A horse's memory is profound.

I feel extremely lucky to have found four great geldings in the past seven years. As with children, I could say that I don't have any favorites, but Barranca will always be my best boy. He is a big chocolate-colored Missouri Fox Trotter, with the kindest eye, a smooth moving, comfortable-gaited horse with a four-beat walk. His forelock ripples over his face and his tail almost sweeps the ground.

While visiting my mother in Scottsdale, Arizona, soon after my father's death, I encountered Barranca in a barn nearby. It was love at first sight. When he saw me coming, he started to prance around his pen, and I was instantly taken. He was recovering from a barbed-wire injury, and I feared that I might be falling for a lame horse with insurmountable problems. But with proper care and chiropractic work, he became the most relaxed and lovely ride. I often feel there is a genuine telepathic communication going on between us.

I had the joy of riding Barranca out West during the winter of this account. During this season I was struggling with my mother's descent into Alzheimer's disease. Mysteriously, during the course of this illness, her once angry, jealous personality was transformed into a sweet and loving presence, making reconciliation possible between us.

But forgiveness is a slow process, and many difficult memories surfaced in the course of writing this book, a process that allowed me to release old hurts and anger. Many of the accounts I share in the italicized portions of this book are part of my struggle to put family problems behind. After sifting through so many scenarios, riding Barranca put me in the moment, which is where I want to live.

In the spring of the year, Barranca came back to the Berkshires of Massachusetts, our primary residence. Rocket, a palomino Tennessee Walker from the Box-Hanging-Three

Ranch in Dubois, Wyoming, became his steady companion. This palomino is never more glorious than when I shampoo his massive mane, which falls equally on either side of his neck. Like most horses, Rocket hates to be left alone. I hope to give him the attention he deserves, so that he doesn't feel compelled to jump out of his stall from a standstill, or leap out of his pasture—quite the escape artist!

Tonka Waken, my Missouri Fox Trotter in Arizona, looks like a strong, solid, Indian pony with a compact body and stud-proud neck. His white-blond forelock falls low on his forehead and he is always eager to get going. I often think of him as my four-wheel-drive vehicle, as he is able to climb almost any incline and actually likes a challenge. An easy keeper, he has the energy and power of a much younger horse. He was born on Valentine's Day.

Peanut, my fourth horse, is everybody's favorite baby. He is the same age as Rocket, but he will always seem like the darling youngster of this equine family. Because of his thin coat, which never seems to grow thick and warm, I chose to leave him in Arizona. With calm amber eyes, he is sweet and gentle. I have had Peanut since he was six months old, and it is a relief to know that he has never been mishandled. I know his history, and there has been nothing traumatic to warp his sense of trust.

On occasion, I rode other horses—in Mexico, Australia, and India. Though these adventures were exciting and new experiences for me, I was always happy to return to Barranca and his gliding gaits. Understanding a horse's soul is more important than mere novelty.

While I love the silence of riding by myself, I also enjoy showing family and friends my favorite spots, exploring new places I wouldn't dare go to alone, riding at dawn or under a full moon, meandering beside the Sonoita Creek where one can wander in and out of the water beneath the carved out bluffs, lying down in a field of wildflowers and dozing off in the sun, or finding a surprising, fresh trail. But the familiar can also be comforting. My familiar horses are my greatest solace, along with my old broken-in saddle and well-worked reins. I hope in the course of this account, you too can take part in the mishaps and delights I have had the privilege to encounter this past year on horseback, lifting us into another realm, purging the daily grumble and allowing our spirits to soar.

ARIZONA

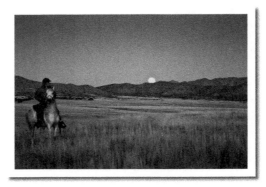

Tonka, Twilight

Blue Moon on the San Rafael

The sun is still high at four o'clock when I drive my horse trailer over the rim of the San Rafael Valley and look out over this glorious prairie grassland. Tightening Tonka's girth, I mount up and head toward Saddle Mountain, bending east along the dirt road toward the headwaters of the Santa Cruz. As the sun begins its descent, light streaks over the rolling valley floor, lighting up the mountains in the distance.

Alone on this great expanse, I worry for a moment about drug runners and illegal transients, but this land seems so gloriously peaceful, I don't want to waste my time picturing dangerous scenarios.

Knowing it will get cold as soon as the sun disappears, I wear a burnt orange parka and gloves. Tonka's thick winter coat is already warming up even though I am not pushing him. I keep stroking his withers, telling him that he is a good boy, and he seems to understand this.

There is something so soothing about riding alone, without the distraction of conversation—just listening to the horse's hooves on the hard-packed road, hearing the swish of water in my plastic bottle strapped to the back of my saddle. Everything is still and subdued. Tonka is a bit wary of his own elongated shadow at first, but then he moves right along with a nice fast walk, standing patiently when I have to dismount to open a cattle gate.

Once I make it to Bog Hole, the headwaters of the Santa Cruz, I check my watch. It is now 5:15 P.M. I believe I should see the moon rise in less than half an hour. This will be a "blue moon," the second full moon this month. I can see my trailer in the distance, a mile or so away.

My neighbors, Al and Judy Blackwell, pass by me in their truck. I have invited their granddaughters to come over on the following morning, New Year's Day, to give them a ride on Peanut, my caramel-and-cream-colored Tennessee Walker. Children love this horse.

Peanut is still recovering from a night out on the range. One night, all three of my boys escaped their corral through a feeble Mexican gate with a flimsy wooden bolt. (I have since added metal closures on either side.)

The next morning, I knew something was wrong as soon as I left the house and didn't see any waiting horses staring over the fence. The open gate confirmed my fears. I only hoped that they had remained inside the federal land that my neighbor, Sonny McQuiston, leases for his cattle, but they knew the terrain well enough, and had found the open passage out to the road. Telltale droppings lay right before the closest cattle guard, where they had stopped and turned, ending up miles away on the Mowry Road near McQuiston's paddock and his one lone horse.

Luckily, none of the three had been seriously injured, but Peanut had cut his fetlock on some barbed wire. I spent the past week doctoring his three-stitch wound, pasting on a pad soaked in antiseptic, and wrapping him with

Christmas-colored, red-and-green wrap, then duct tape. The little pad inevitably fell out during the night, so I was now simply spraying his sore with antiseptic. *There is always something happening with horses.*

A month ago, when I trailered Barranca up to the San Rafael alone, he rode out nicely as always, but when I loaded him back into the trailer and retreated to shut the door, he broke free, jumped out and ran off with his tether flying. I felt stupid—not having tied a proper cowboy knot, and helpless, for out on this wide open range I had no hope of catching him on foot. All I could think of was more barbed wire and dangerous cattle guards.

Panicked, I immediately called my husband Mason on my cell phone. He drove out, and we passed each other on the road as I pulled the empty trailer back home to pick up Tonka, thinking I might be able to catch Barranca on horseback before he got into trouble. By the time I returned with Tonka in tow, Mason was standing by the side of the road with Barranca tied to an oak tree. Two helpful men had caught my renegade and secured him. People take care of each other out here, and I was extremely grateful. Shaken, Barranca was quick to join his equine companion, and I had escaped a close disaster.

This past year streams through my mind as I ride back up the darkening valley. I think of my mother, descending into Alzheimer's and wonder where this disease will take her. Her days are now only barely lit, as if she too is waiting in semi-darkness.

I still detect no moon glow, and wonder if my calculations have been wrong. But just before I reach the dirt road that crosses the valley floor, I look to my left and catch the enormous upper lip of the golden saucer ascending above the mountains. Quickly, it rises, magnified in size, and a thrill goes through me—just seeing it makes me let out a *whoop* as I canter up the incline. Suddenly the moon is there in full form, balanced on the mountain line and rising surely, revealing its golden appearance as it continues to ascend, shedding its light on the last of the old year and the beginning of the next.

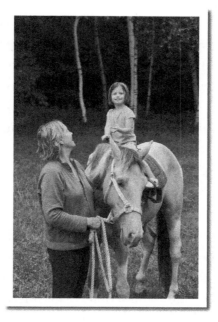

Laura and Lucy

Rough Riders in the Making

As planned, my neighbors bring their two little girls over to the house at 10:30 A.M. The horses have already been fed, and I've haltered Peanut. Both girls are wearing colorful bike helmets, and my four-year-old goddaughter, Lucy, comes out to watch, somewhat in awe of these older children.

Ashley, aged nine, has close-cropped hair. She has just undergone a non-malignant brain tumor operation. What an ordeal for a small child. She is calm and reserved, while her six-year-old sister is wild and enthusiastic. Well, she was named "Haley" after all. She is eager to help brush Peanut, watching me pick his hooves, dashing here and there.

Ashley stands on the mounting block and manages to hoist herself into the saddle. We walk down the dirt drive all the way out to the road. I am happy to give these girls a chance to ride. Lucy is all eyes, and though she just rode Peanut yesterday with a parent on either side, today she declines. So Haley the comet gets a turn in her purple helmet. The girls discuss their favorite colors, and Lucy pipes up, "I like *maroon!*"

Haley would like to trot or even canter, but I am leading, and Peanut is taking his time. I tell her that I think she has "the horse bug," and that she will become a real rider. "You can even ride with me in a few years," I say.

Sharing my riding life with these girls, I am reminded of all I received in my childhood. I was passionate about horses from an early age, strapped into the saddle by the time I was two. As a child, I found the greatest times of togetherness riding alone with my father. Off through the open fields of Wisconsin—off into the dairy wind.

Out on the trail we were free, part of nature, at one with our horses and each other, embraced by the deep green foliage of the Prime Woods or the Nashotah Mission forest, alert to holes when we galloped the trolley track, whisking the heads and rumps of our mounts, so they knew we were not so unlike them.

After putting Peanut away, the three little girls explore the courtyard and all the secret hiding places—the gate that leads to the back garden and the pathway up to the mesa. Haley's mother has to keep telling her younger daughter to slow down, be careful, *stop*, to not grab everything, but it falls on deaf ears. She is dealing with a comet, after all, a rough rider in the making.

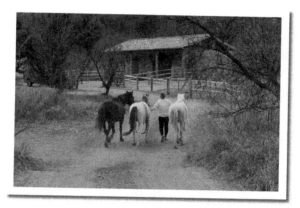

Bringing the Horses In

Snow on the Road

This morning looks like it will warm up quickly, and I decide to trailer Barranca up to Flux Canyon. There are still remnants of snow here from the big storm ten days ago. We climb the hill from Mowry Road, and begin the descent on the other side of the ridge. My Standard Poodles, Bali and Cello, are with me today, padding along in tandem. There is nothing nicer than riding out on a good, steady horse with attentive dogs by your side.

Maybe this isn't snow, but a strange white powder—calcium, gypsum, alum? There has been a lot of exploratory mining going on in these hills recently. It seems tragic to disturb the peaceful grandeur of these mountains just to collect copper, silver, or manganese for fiscal gain. But today it is amazingly quiet. I feel like I am the only one enjoying this great expanse. Nobody else is out here, *just me and the drug runners.*

Continuing on down the slope, I can see Mount Wrightson poking up in the distance behind Red Mountain's muscular yet feminine form. Up ahead there's a huge grey outcropping I like to think of as "Rhino Rock"—so different from the rest of the iron-rich, red-colored mountains. I wonder about this landscape, its geologic history—what it is made of, when it was formed.

A deer bounds away up the slope, and I am aware that mountain lions are becoming more of a presence. Recently a friend saw three grown lions crossing Harshaw Creek Road just a hundred feet from our driveway. Surely there are enough deer around to satisfy these carnivores, but still it worries me. I imagine seeing a big cat, and wonder what I would do to scare it away. Would it be interested in my dogs, trotting along so faithfully?

I have forgotten my water bottle and am now very thirsty. Barranca stops to sample various puddles—some of which are probably filled with iron or sulphur or worse. Who knows what elements the mining has disturbed? The proposed Wildcat Mine is planning a massive 150-acre open pit with trucks running down Harshaw Road every eight minutes. I wonder how the Forest Service, which is supposedly the steward of our public land, can let this happen? Who knows what this operation will do to our already compromised water, not to mention the rest of the local ecology?

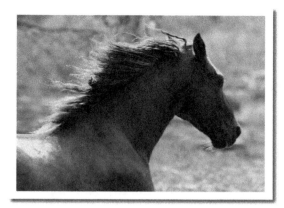

Barranca on the Move

Sisters in the Saddle

My sister Cia arrives today with Mom and Wanda, our mother's caregiver. Mom's Alzheimer's has clearly progressed. After greeting me, she asks, "Whose house is this? Have I been here before?" though she has visited me three times since November. Her mind is like a Teflon pan—everything sliding right off. Mysteriously, this disease—so terrible in many ways—has allowed her to forget many of the conflicts of our past and has made her a much nicer person.

The beds are all made, and supper composed, so I urge my sister to come out and ride with me. I am willing to give her my best boy, Barranca, though she is somewhat wary due to her last ride here a couple of years ago, when a friend's horse dumped her in the wash.

As we head out, I suggest that we try to focus on riding, and not talk too much, for I have noticed when riding with groups of women—and surely I am as much to blame as my companions—there is an almost compulsive need to communicate. Often a ride of three or four can be a cacophony, close to distracting.

It is nice to be comfortable enough with a riding partner (like I am with my cousin Helen) to not have to talk constantly. But Cia and I have a lot of catching up to do. We are both concerned about our mother—her medications, her bruising, her balance, and of course, her mental state.

We proceed up a very steep hill where Cia can get a full view of the mountains. It pleases me to hear her awed response to this expansive desert landscape.

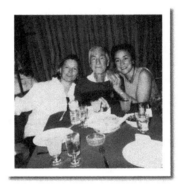

La Roca

Cia would often visit me here in Arizona, bringing our ailing father down from Scottsdale. Since I was not welcome at my mother's house for the past few years, this was the easiest way for me to see them, and I always looked forward to their company.

On his last visit to Patagonia, we took Popi across the border to La Roca, in Nogales, Mexico. But did we push him too far, ordering chicken mole, letting him drink margaritas, forbidden in terms of his therapy? We hired mariachis to play

"Rancho Grande" and had our photo taken together, one adoring daughter on either side. At the time, we didn't realize that this would be our last meal together.

Popi's story is a big part of this narrative, for he played a major role in the conflict between my mother and me. I cannot really understand my mother or the dynamic between us, without looking at our family as a whole.

As children, we would wait for our father to come home, anticipating his return. Mom would dress up every night like a good fifties wife, meeting him at the door with a hug and a kiss. They would have cocktails, usually a glass of sherry in the library, and I would fiddle with the combination on his caramel-brown briefcase, 3-9-5, until it popped open, exposing his gargantuan legal files.

He was a big important man, not only to me, but to that other world of business. Yet I could see he often drifted in a daze. I was like him, both in temperament and looks, big-boned, hazel-eyed, with a naughty sense of humor. Popi liked to have a good time and his circle of friends embraced him. He liked to include anyone and everyone, while my mother wanted to keep everybody out. She wanted him all to herself.

On those nights when we ate together around the formal dining room table, it was a chance to teach us manners, but with milk spilling down the mahogany cracks, my jumping up and down, David's antics, Cia's diabetes, George's baiting, and Popi's amusement by it all, how could our mother maintain a civilized dinner? She often ended up in tears.

I didn't realize that what was bothering her was something more important than manners. I remember her sometimes sitting there in silence, barely picking at her food. Even if we asked her a question, she would not speak. One cannot say the unthinkable.

But when they went out in the evening, it was a different mood. Popi would be all dressed up in seal-like-sleekness, with flat pearl studs running up his crisp looking shirt. His gloves were immense and lined with real cashmere. His ring was a garnet signet ring. The emblem on that impressed me. Now I wonder—where did that ring go? Did he give it to one of his "friends"? And how glamorous she looked on the way to the opera or symphony, her hair done to perfection, her jewelry and dress so elegant. She would walk away on his arm with such grace.

But I felt a pang of abandonment when they left me at home with my siblings, all of us together in the breakfast nook, inspecting eggs for that dreaded clot of blood, or eating creamed tuna fish in fried potato baskets as our elegant parents slid past us, wishing us all a most fragrant goodnight.

I liked the roughness of my father's cheek on the weekends, his long yellow legal pads, and his peculiar print-script, the cardboard embedded in his freshly cleaned shirts—which I collected for my writing and artwork—his impressive china dog collection, which I emulated with my own assortment of horses. He had a compulsion to see things clean and neat—Saturday morning room inspection, mad polisher of shoes. He would lead wild dashes in the airport, hollering for attention, "Run! RUN!!!" Just-making-it-without-one-minute-to-spare was his favored method for takeoff. To him, creating anxiety was part of the program, though he thought it all a big joke.

I can't quite picture our mother running in her narrow skirt and two-toned heels. Once Popi got to the gate, huffing and puffing, perhaps he managed to convince the stewardess to hold the plane until our mother sauntered up, southern style. I think he really liked her complaints, which he pretended not to hear, making her even madder. He liked playing the part of "bad boy," doing exactly as he wanted, riling her up.

It was only after a hard week's work that he finally seemed utterly spent. Then he was ready to get down on the dark red carpet and let me ride his back, bouncing before the fire, giving me a good buck.

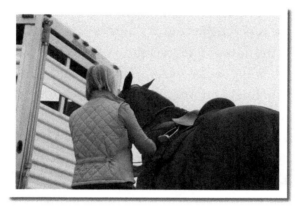

Ready to Load

Back Wash

Cynthia Carlisi is coming over to give Mom a massage today, but my horse trailer blocks Cynthia's arrival, and Barranca is balking again, not wanting to load. I'm getting really tired of this. Cynthia gives her free advice—*Don't use food or treats to entice a horse into a trailer.* I agree, but often opt for the easier way out—a handful of grain or a carrot, though neither is helping today.

Barranca keeps veering off to the side, and I try backing him up, as Les Spath did when he came to train Barranca in Massachusetts. Les took his time and was clearly the boss. If Barranca wouldn't load, he had to back up. Most horses soon learn that it is easier to go forward.

But now there is way too much nervous energy all around and perhaps Barranca is picking up on that. Finally, with Cynthia clucking from behind, Barranca makes his move and loads. I close the divider and Tonka hops in, then Cia and I drive up the washboard-rough road and disembark in front of the Hale Ranch, with its graceful meadow slopes. It reminds me of some turn-of-the-century homestead with its old wood-and-tin outbuildings and mesquite stick corral.

After warming the horses up, I suggest that we canter to the top of an incline. I go first, loping gently, but I hear a rustle in the bushes behind me and then a *yelp* from my sister. Barranca has shied, unusual for him. I can see that she has lost her stirrup and is unbalanced, but at least she stays in the saddle. "Did something spook him?" She doesn't know, but I don't want to see my sister take another fall, so I suggest that we take it easy.

Tonka feels like quite a handful today. He keeps throwing his head up and down, acting competitive—he hates to have Barranca ahead of him, especially when we canter. Barranca, always the equine gentleman, allows the unruly Tonka to go before him. Sometimes when Tonka acts out like this, I am reminded of a misbehaving child, and how that reflects poorly on the parents. Most likely I only have myself to blame for Tonka's faults.

That night we set up a fire in the living room and turn the lights low. Our mother is in an excellent mood—so happy to be visiting, to be here with us both. The glowing hearth makes her feel at home, for she always had a passion for building a fire.

Every night before dinner Mom would crush newspaper and stuff it beneath the logs in the living room. The fire flared up beneath a painted sea scene that hung above the mantel where waves were caught in an eternal crash—far from our Midwestern landscape.

On occasion, we would set up those flimsy TV-dinner trays and watch the fire for entertainment. My older brother, George, and I would take turns throwing a special chemical powder onto the blaze, creating tongues of blue and green, while Cia and David, sprawled on the floor in their footsie pajamas. Chipper, our Boxer, lay asleep on the floor. I rubbed his floppy ears.

Once in a while after dinner, if our father was in the mood, he would clap his hands together and ask if we'd like a story. In silent agreement we would huddle together on the dark red carpet and watch the fire as it transformed his kind, attractive face into something almost scary, grotesque. We didn't have to ask what he was going to read. It was always the same story: "Bluebeard."

Our mother didn't stay to listen to Popi's favorite fairytale. She retreated to the kitchen to clean up the Formica-countered kitchen with its checkered floor, everything nice and orderly, the stay-a-bed stew put away in its Pyrex container, the budgie-bird tray swept clean. Our mother had a firm idea of what the perfect fifties family was supposed to be like and it included bedtimes, table manners, and nightly prayers.

"Open them all; go into each and every one of them," our father read, "except that little closet which I forbid you...."

As the four of us children heeded this warning, delivered by our father's scariest voice, we would shudder in anticipation. I'd put a hand on Chipper's dignified head, hoping he would protect me. My other hand would slip through the opening in the mahogany coffee table, needing something to hang onto. Or I'd play with the empty, silver humidor, which retained the delicious scent of tobacco—open-shut, open-shut.

"She then took the little key, and opened it, trembling," our father continued, excited by the terrible tension of the story. "At first she could not see anything plainly, but after some moments, she began to perceive that the floor was all covered with clotted blood, on which lay the bodies of several dead women, ranged against the walls."

In the story the key fell from her hands into a pool of blood. We all knew that the stain would betray her. Bluebeard would know that she knew!

The waves above the fireplace should have sprung into life at that point in the story, crashing against the shore, washing the key with its magical waters. But my father read on in a tone of great warning, as if we too must always obey and never violate the sanctity of the closet.

Luckily, Bluebeard's wife had a younger sister, who ran to the top of the tower to look out for their brothers. LO! There in the distance came the rescuers riding—two brothers racing across the desert, approaching in a cloud of dust! I liked this part of the story—riders coming to the rescue. I wondered if my own two brothers would be as valiant.

In the story, the brothers arrived just in time, as Bluebeard took hold of the young wife's hair and prepared to strike off her head. Before he had a chance, the brothers sprang up the steps and ran their swords through the old man's body, and all four happy siblings were united.

After that cheery ending, it was time to kiss our parents goodnight, then trot upstairs, where we could say the Lord's Prayer and have "Sweet Dreams." No wonder I had recurring nightmares.

Now Mom rests in the corner of our big French-blue sofa, propped up by pillows, sipping her *faux Bellini*—bubbly water and pomegranate juice—served in an elegant champagne flute. I call her, "My Baby Mama," and she smiles back, saying sweetly, "My two little girls." Not so little, I think.

It is hard to imagine our mother dying. She has always had such a strong constitution and an almost manic energy. I could see her dwindling life going on and on, slowly rolling downhill into that murky region of Alzheimer's land, the mind giving up, but the body resisting.

Six years ago my relationship with her was so different. Even now, I am still finding my way back to the mother who'd rejected me out of misplaced jealousy and anger.

On the morning of my father's death, my mother called our house eight times telling me NOT to come to Scottsdale—I was not wanted, my father was fine, I was not allowed in intensive care, he could not be disturbed, he was stable, no problem, he needed to rest, I would only be in the way.

My husband Mason thought that I should wait and respect my mother's wishes. But I had respected those wishes for the past several months, staying away, even though we were living only three hours south in the little town of Patagonia. When I wanted to visit my father in his failing state, I was told, "Why don't you wait until you're asked, Laura?"

But my older brother, George, sensed the pressure of time. "Dad might not make it through the weekend." This shocked me. I didn't believe it, but I called the Mayo Clinic to check on my father's condition. "Is it true that he can't be disturbed?"

The nurse said, "He's expecting you."

Luckily I had my cell phone and was able to get directions as I entered Phoenix. When I spotted the clinic across the barren field, it looked like an enormous jack-in-the-box, a monument to illness.

I dashed up to intensive care where a doctor greeted me at the security door, escorting me to a windowless anteroom. "About twenty minutes ago," the kindly doctor began, very tentative, not knowing how I would take this, "your father seemed stable. We thought he was doing well."

Just minutes before my arrival, Popi had been talking and joking with his doctors, and then suddenly something changed. Part of him had slipped away. I took this news in blankly.

The doctor led me to a nearby room where Popi was laid out on a table, tipped at a disconcerting angle, so that his head was lower than his feet. He was hooked up to various machines with flashing, changing numbers. Numerous doctors stood in a semi-circle by his bed—one Indian doctor wore a turban and held a fist to his mouth. It was as if representatives of healing from all over the globe had flown in to be in attendance. They were silent, respectful, observing their patient.

I went down on my knees, taking his hand. "Dad," I said, "I'm here. It's Laura." His face looked so handsome, peaceful.

No response.

Mom was at home in bed. She had just received a phone call, telling her to come.

Later she told us that just moments before her phone rang, a bobcat slowly sauntered past her bedroom window, right next to the huge plate glass, peering in. I couldn't help but think that my father, the prankster, had chosen the body of a bobcat to tease her, to make his last farewell, all the while enjoying the fun of startling my mother out of bed.

But now it was as if I was talking by cell phone, not knowing if we were still connected. The circle of doctors slipped away. Only one remained. "What do those numbers mean?" I asked. They were steadily falling from 113, to 110, 98, 97...

"His heart is slowing down."

"Shouldn't we try to keep him alive until my mother gets here?"

The doctor responded, "Just this morning, your father requested no heroic measures."

I nodded.

Popi's hand was still warm, still alive, so I whispered the Lord's Prayer and told him how much we all loved him, how he had been the very best father, that we would take care of Mom and his horses. "Go, Dad, go. Don't hold on. It's okay. You know that we love you very, very much."

And then just as easily as a fountain clicks off from its steadily rising and falling motion, the water of his life became still. Peacefully silent, without any pain or even a gasp, as simple as that, it was over. The numbers rested at zero.

Then my mother walked in. The first words out of her mouth were, "What are you doing here? I told you not to come!" followed by a weeping intake of breath, as she went to him, her husband.

As I left the room, Wanda, my parents' housekeeper for over twenty years, was backing away. "What are we going to do now?" She didn't know how she would function without his kindly protection.

She went on to tell me how close my parents had been during those final weeks. But he had been tending to her, and no one had been looking out for him, as he didn't like having anyone hovering over him. After all, he had spent most of his life trying to escape "The Mother," and he had done a fine job—he had escaped us all, for good.

When I went back into the room a few minutes later, Mom was still whimpering. I sat down on the edge of the bed beside his body and said to her, "Our relationship is going to be different now."

She answered simply, "Yes."

And then, it was as if some dark tattered veil fell from her shoulders, the shroud she had worn for him, like a protective cloth that deflected attention away from his secret life. It was *an instant of transformation that I could barely trust, though the change itself was visceral. She no longer seemed to hate me. She had become like a child, needing me, wanting me to stay with her, but was the rivalry really over? Were we allies now in death?*

Sitting together now in our living room, the fire settles down into embers, and my sister and I start getting silly, laughing over the blog I tried to create for this book last fall.

"The day I wrote my first entry, I was going down this flat dirt road—there were no holes or ruts or anything— and Rocket just fell down, on TOP of me!" We all find this hilarious. "And then the next day when I searched the Internet, I couldn't even find my own blog!"

At last we can laugh together.

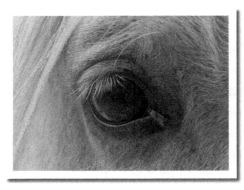

Tonka's Eye

You Don't See Them, but They See You

Riding Barranca beneath the big-boned sycamores that line Harshaw Creek, a few leaves left clattering, little golden balls dangle like leftover Christmas decorations. Picking our way around thorny mesquite, I break branches where necessary, so that each time I come this way there will be less chance of getting clawed.

In Massachusetts, falling off is not such a threat. The earth is sodden, and the trails often soft with mud. But here in the desert the ground is like cement, the climate harsh, trees rough and ready to get you. Old mesquite breaks brittle in my hands. Riding out onto the sand of the wash feels safer, and I let Barranca canter. He has a lovely fast walk and a graceful, smooth lope, but he is still somewhat wary of cattle.

Climbing up an extremely rocky hillside, he keeps trying to turn toward home, but I insist, firmly, and he goes on. Not far away, there is a little turn out, and I see that many transients have come through here. There is a scattering of plastic bottles, black-washed for camouflage, discarded clothing, toilet paper stuck in crannies, a little cave with a sleeping ledge, opened tins of food, the remnants of a fire for cooking or warmth.

One border patrol friend, Danny Cantou, said, "You don't see them, but they see you." Danny informed me that they recently captured five men with semiautomatics in a cave right above one of the gates I open to go toward the Hale homestead. Last year I found six, fifty-pound bales of marijuana less than a mile from our house, and more recently a truck with 1,850 pounds of grass was apprehended on our small road. In response, the border patrol began setting up sensors along various footpaths—one of which is a favorite riding trail.

When I get home, I give Barranca a bath with warm hose water, then work some Cowboy Magic conditioner into his tail and proceed to comb out the snarls. I've heard that horses are quite proud of their tails, and his is exceptionally long and thick, almost sweeping the ground. The dark brown strands are streaked with gold, just like his fetlocks. I think he likes the feel of his dust-free hide, the sensation of my hands separating the strands of his magnificent banner.

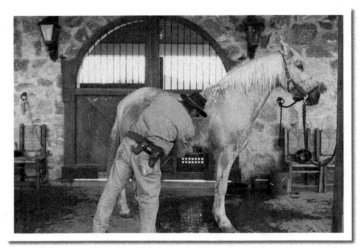

Washing Tonka

Blackwell Canyon

I decide to take Barranca out today, and put my friend, Phil Caputo, on Tonka. For the most part I am the only one who has ridden Barranca these past three years, and he has responded well to my consistency, but now, too often, I am tempted to let others ride him because he is the easiest horse with the best gaits. I know Tonka is a bit of a challenge, but Phil is a trooper.

I call my neighbor, Al Blackwell, and tell him that we are going to ride through his ranch on our way up the canyon. The Blackwells are unusually good neighbors, and let me keep my horses in their stone corral before we had our own barn. Twice a day I made the one-mile drive down Harshaw Creek to feed, and the Blackwells never made me feel like I was violating their privacy. Judy would go out and sit in her chair and watch the horses, getting so much pleasure from just seeing them there. I prefer having my boys at home now, but still miss the old, stone corral and adobe outbuildings nestled in at the foot of Indianhead Mountain.

Dismounting, we walk the horses under the Blackwell's open-air barn and let ourselves out through the back gate. I tighten Phil's girth and adjust his stirrups. He wears a Smith & Wesson pistol at his waist, and somehow that gives me some assurance as we head up this well-known drug-runners' trail. I have ridden this way numerous times and am now more familiar with the route, though it's always a bit tricky starting out until we find the well-trodden path that runs in and out of the wash. Along the way, through this intimate, wind-protected canyon, we note the scattered water bottles, abandoned backpacks, and other transient debris.

Recently, I came upon Danny Cantou's wife, Summer, who was patrolling this trail with another officer. Summer used to ride with the mounted border patrol. She once told me that she was able to contain a large group of illegals by telling them she was riding an attack horse, and the first one who ran would get trampled. Summer was a beautiful, fearless young woman who was also a champion kickboxer and award-winning marksman—shooting targets at a full gallop. But I was shocked to see that her partner was holding a fifteen-pound AK-47.

"You really should be armed out here," she told me.

Well, at least Phil had a gun, though we both knew it would do little to help us if we ran into a bunch of thugs. Gangs from Tucson were coming down to raid the poor guys who did the hauling from Mexico. These "mules" were more apt to be armed now in an attempt to protect their contraband, so violence was increasing. Phil's theory was that if you wore a gun, you had to be prepared to use it, and if you used it, you had to be prepared to kill. I was not prepared to do that.

Determined to go as far as we can, we have packed our lunches and tucked them into our saddlebags. This is a beautiful and varied canyon, but a bit like a roller-coaster ride, up and down, dodging mesquite, leaping into the wash and back out. We maneuver along the single-file trail that the horses remember better than we do. Horses have a great sense of direction, perfect memories for what they have and have not seen before—even a new fallen tree can be cause for alarm.

Phil has a low deep voice, so it is easy to hear him talk as we ride. Stopping to open various cattle gates, I hop off, for I can easily mount and dismount, while he has sustained several injuries from various journalistic assignments in the Middle East. Years ago he won a Pulitzer Prize for investigative journalism, but he doesn't like to dwell on his past achievements. He's more concerned about the synopsis for his next book, still in the mulling stage. He describes how hemmed in he feels by having to write out a plot line for his publisher before they will approve the book. Writers like to allow a story to unfold, just as we like to discover where we're going when entering new riding territory.

We come to the familiar hillside of red gravel where the path is cut into the mountain. I usually turn around at this point, but now I open another gate and we ride on, wondering where we are headed. Are we riding toward Meadow Valley or north through the Canelo Hills?

We approach a rather treacherous stretch of smooth, black rock that is very slippery. I assume it is sedimentary since it is within the wash, but we manage to get over it, climbing up the steep parts and sliding back down into the sand of the riverbed, happily surprised to see a little creek running alongside the trail here. We follow it for a mile or so, but when we come to yet another cattle barrier, one that looks like it would be too difficult to dismantle, we decide to stop and break for lunch.

I hold both horses while Phil sits in the sand and eats his sandwich and Fritos. I try giving the horses a couple of chips but they are not sure about the crunchy texture of this junk food. They're more interested in splitting Phil's apple core.

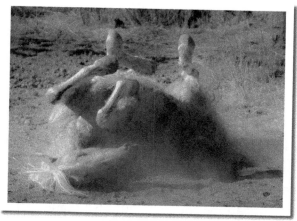

Bagna de Terra

Tightening up Barranca's girth after our rest stop, I hold the opposite stirrup on Phil's saddle as he mounts. Tonka seems overly eager, throwing his head and breaking into a canter every chance he gets. What is his problem?

By the time we return to the barn, we see that we've been out for almost five hours. We figure we must have ridden about twelve miles over some fairly rough territory. I want to give the horses a bath, and collect two pails of warm water from the house. We sponge them down, and curry them, before they proceed to ruin our work, taking their *bagna de terra* out in the corral.

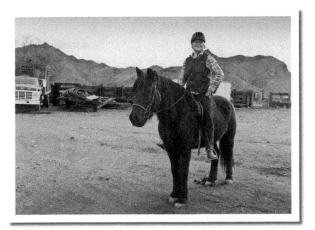

El Chapo

Such a Sucker

Why am I such a sucker for almost every available horse I see? I just talked to Ian Wingfield, who inherited his uncle's ranch in Amado on the Tubac side of the Santa Ritas. Not only did he receive this adobe fortress, but also some cattle and six horses, one of which is supposedly a small Friesian. Is there such a thing as a *small* Friesian? Of course, I am curious to see this horse, eager to see it, imagining its long black mane blowing in the wind.

Agua Caliente was once a huge working ranch started by Ian's grandfather, but the family sold off most of the land, and now only this section remains. Ian, Mason, and I plan on meeting at the ranch around nine in the morning. I wake before the alarm goes off in order to feed my horses and walk them across the road to their pasture. Then I pile the car with saddle, pad, bridles, halters, currycombs, and leads. I want to try to ride this little Friesian and assess his potential, though he might not have been ridden in some time.

I know what a Friesian should look like, so I'm a bit surprised to see El Chapo (the short one), who only stands about 14 hands. (With horses, four inches equals a "hand.") He is black with the traditional full mane, but he has very few "feathers" on his fetlocks. Perhaps he is a crossbreed. His temperament is calm and sweet, and he is easy to catch and halter. I put Barranca's dressage saddle on him, and the stirrups look absurdly long. He takes the bit, and I adjust the bridle. He doesn't seem to mind much.

No one has any idea if this horse has ever been ridden. So I strap on my hard hat and lead the little Friesian around the yard. He follows me like a docile doggie, quite endearing. He is easy to mount, so close to the ground, yet he does not seem used to the bit. El Chapo walks out nicely enough and has a great big trot. I need to post and realize how I have become used to the flat gaits of my walking horses. He doesn't seem to understand my request for a canter. Perhaps he was never trained to the saddle, but with his quiet nature I assume he could become a nice child's horse.

Ian is very enthusiastic about his ranch and his excitement is infectious. Even though his uncle was an eccentric recluse, they had a nice connection. Geoff Wingfield, Ian's uncle, had been a self-made archeologist, and after I ride El Chapo around the yard, Ian takes me through his uncle's garrison-style dwelling. It feels like something from another era. Every window has a place to set one's rifle, just like the old Wild West. The gates are narrow, and the plank steps up to the tower are short and steep. The thought was that if one was attacked, it would take more time for the enemy to get up those steps.

In the bedroom, where his uncle died not long ago, there is a metal bed frame without a mattress and a nice old armoire. "He had his hands crossed over his chest," Ian says, "so we assumed it was a heart attack." There are piles of old family photographs, boxes of arrowheads and cabinets of Indian pottery—like a mini-museum. Ian seems like he will be the perfect family curator.

I tell him that I would be willing to take El Chapo on trial, but what with hay, feed, shoeing, and vetting, the initial price is only part of the expense involved. Plus, I already have my hands full.

"What do you need a miniature draft horse for?" Phil asks me later, and I have to respond—"Good question!"

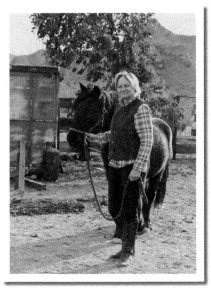

Not Ready to Go

Spurs of the Moment

I decide to make the drive back to Amado to pick up El Chapo. No one else will be at the ranch, but Ian tells me which gates to open, and I am confident about going alone with my two Standard Poodles, Bali and Cello.

At the ranch, I halter El Chapo, leaving the dogs in the truck, as there is a vicious sounding Pit Bull barking behind the fence to the house. I have brought along a good supply of apples and carrots, and El Chapo is interested in the treats, but when it comes to the trailer, he only puts his two front feet in, then immediately backs out, repeating this stunt over and over.

Barranca behaved the same way when Les Spath tried to load him in Massachusetts, and I knew I had to be patient and encouraging, backing him up when he refuses to enter. But it is not easy backing up a reluctant, hefty pony, not used to going in reverse. I try again to entice him, but like most ponies he is wily and stretches out his neck to get what he can without committing himself to the trailer. I am getting hot and take off my outer shirt. I don't know why I imagined this would be easy. The other horses watch with interest from inside their corral. Do they think this is funny? Do they wonder where El Chapo is going? Or do they even care? Life in a bare paddock must be boring, and the other horses seem mildly entertained by our antics.

I hate for this little guy to get the best of me, but I am running out of patience. Finally, he loads, all four feet, but instead of standing by him calmly, congratulating him as I should, I tie his lead rope and make a move to close the divider. He freaks out, pulling back as if his survival depends on it. Not a proper "unload." Now I have one broken halter that I tie around his neck and El Chapo is unnerved. I try scooping out some pellets from the can in the shed and entice him with that, but to no avail.

I even try placing a rope around the back of his butt, pulling him forward, but he ducks under, off to the side.

I try a few encouraging taps on his rear to get him going, but he seems insensitive, confused, and I don't want to upset him further. So, after two hours of effort, I give up. What else can I do at this point? In any case, I'm not sure if I want another difficult loader.

I remember the old black groom, Pinky, who once tried to load my horse, Zucchero. The horse was reluctant, balking, so Pinky took a crop and jammed it up the horse's ass. Zucchero sprang into the trailer. I am not about to imitate that move, but I'm sure if Les Spath was on hand, he would get El Chapo loaded.

Later that day, Ian checks in by email, saying that he found out that El Chapo is not a Friesian but a twelve-year-old Welsh pony. Twelve is not old for this breed.

My son's New Forest pony lived to a ripe old age. When Ayler was in third grade, I bought Star for his birthday. When Ayler awoke, a used English saddle was sitting on the footboard of his bed, and his black pony was out in the corral. We had five years of glorious rides together. The two of us would often go down trails holding hands, or we'd gallop up dirt roads and explore new territory, sometimes getting chased by land owners. *What a time.*

But when Ayler went into eighth grade, his interest in team sports took over, so we gave Star away to a family with several little girls who loved this able yet aging pony. Later, we found out that after the girls had outgrown Star, the pony was returned to the original owner, who now had her own daughter, and Star was almost forty!

So a twelve-year-old Welsh sounds like a youngster. He could still have years ahead of him. Maybe the trouble with this pony is his name, "El Chapo," the nickname of Mexico's most wanted fugitive, Joaquin Guzman, head of the Sinaloa drug cartel, a mean and evil dude. Maybe the pony needs a gentle and obedient name, like *El Guapo*, handsome guy. Names often influence human personality, so why shouldn't the same be true for horses?

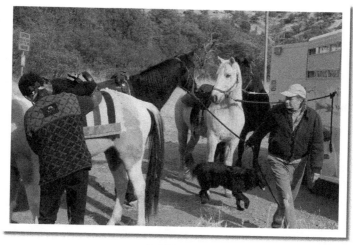

Saddling Up

Ladies Trail Lunch

My good friend, the photographer Donna DeMari, is here for a visit. I show her my morning routine of haying, mucking, graining, grooming, and it is nice to have her help. The rain seems to be holding off, and I wonder how many more days we'll have before the predicted deluge.

This morning Helen is picking up Phil's wife, Leslie Ware, in town and bringing her horse Bendajo over to ride with mine. I am letting Donna ride Barranca as I know he will put her at ease. While the clouds are building, the sun comes and goes, perfect sweater weather, and a good day for a lunch ride.

The four horses feel like a herd moving out, going nicely up the hill toward Humboldt Canyon, but when we begin to canter, Tonka and Barranca jockey for lead position.

Riding into the canyon, we anthropomorphize various tall standing rocks—one looks just like a Gila Monster with his eye on a little stone chipmunk across the way. This is a beautiful conifer-laden canyon with rock outcroppings of chartreuse and burnt amber. We spot a Madonna plaque high on the canyon wall, just outside a small cave that protects a statue of Our Lady of Guadalupe. Someday I'll bring my tennis shoes and climb up there to have a look, but today we're all wearing leather boots.

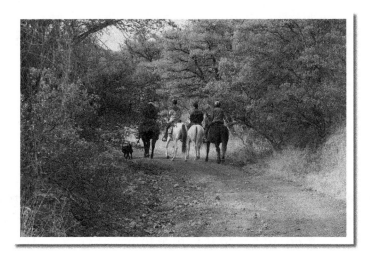

Riding Out

Last May, Mason and I drove the Ford pickup to the end of Humboldt Canyon to celebrate our anniversary. I brought along a picnic, as well as a nice bottle of Australian Shiraz that my son, Clovis, had sent from Sydney. Maybe it was the bumpy road that addled my brain, or perhaps I drank the wine too fast, but I got the spins, and had to walk back out, following Mason in the truck. The road never felt bumpy on horseback for some reason. Do horses have better shocks?

Today, three of us are protected by helmets, but Helen is only wearing a baseball cap. This concerns me because several years ago she survived a terrible fall from a friend's horse, bashing her head on a gravel road, ending up in a coma for over a week. But people out West rarely wear hard hats, as if they're defying the possibility of an accident, defying gravity, so to speak.

We ride on beside a little stream that trickles down through the canyon, and the dogs get a chance to drink. I ask Helen why she didn't bring her Pit Bull, Brindie, and Helen admits, "I can't stand the sound of her breathing."

At the end of this rolling trail, stiff green grass grows around a burbling spring that is always continually flowing. We loosen the horses' girths, take off their bridles, and tie them up before settling down for lunch. I sit on a felled pine tree to eat and the sap sticks to the seat of my breeches. Once mounted, I find that I'm stuck to the saddle, so that when I stand in my stirrups, it sounds like ripping Velcro.

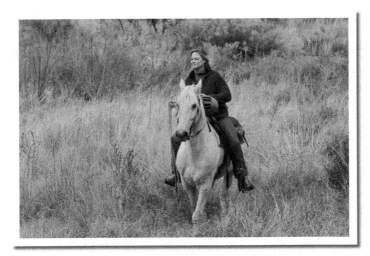

Laura on Tonka

Cold Crotches

It's a brand new day—Donna and I saddle up early and head down the road to Blackwell Canyon. Though it is a very rough path, Donna is entranced by the intimate landscape, saying how she likes the grey light. A photographer always sees things differently. Now it looks like it is about to rain, but I think it might hold off. It seems like this storm is all anyone can talk about—we need winter rain so badly.

Donna is having a good time on my best boy, but I am beginning to miss him, eager to let him know I have not forsaken him. Maybe I'll go back to reclaiming him as *my one and only*. I don't share my husband, so why loan out my favorite horse?

I decide to turn back before we hit a steep, slick patch of rock, as the sky now looks forbidding. As we turn, we can see thin veils of cloud descending over Red Mountain. Up above, the grey mammatus clouds have taken on the appearance of Pillsbury dough buns stuck together. Then the rain starts falling—*brrrrrr*—slashing down at an angle.

Of course, the horses are excited by this strange weather. The wet earthy smell on the once dusty path is delicious, nothing like rain dampening the desert. But then, it turns into tiny pellets of hail. We are moving fast, our pants getting soaked in the saddle, sitting in puddles of icy water—wet crotches! All very invigorating, I'm sure, when we know there will be a hot steam shower waiting for us at home.

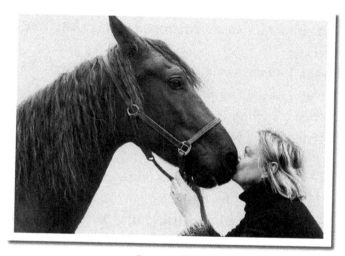

Barranca Boy

Etchings in the Wash

Yesterday's snow chill is still in the air, though the scant white covering has already melted. The short-lived drama of the running wash has passed, and the sloppy road is firm again. It's been a week since I've ridden Barranca, so I saddle him up, and we head down Harshaw Creek toward the Turner's

Ranch about three miles away. I rarely go this way because there are four cattle guards and gates that I have to open, but Barranca stands nicely as I open and close each one. I have both dogs with me today. They can drink from the small, winding creek that runs through the canyon here, dodging the cattle that graze down below.

I remember when Mason and I were looking at land out on the San Rafael Valley and my parents came down from Scottsdale to consider it with us. My mother's response was, "Who would want to build in this godforsaken place? You should look for land along that small dirt road by the creek. That would be perfect."

Though I was disappointed that she didn't appreciate the vast expanse of the San Rafael Valley, I knew she had a point. We ended up buying ten acres at the end of Harshaw Creek and now see it as a preferable location.

One day years ago, when I was taking the dogs for a walk, I came upon a horrible sight here—a huge pile of young cow carcasses on the road. A cattle transport truck had tipped over the edge at one of the sharper turns, landing in the stream below. Most of the calves had died on impact and had to be lifted out with a front-end loader. Why the driver had taken the right hand turn onto this small dirt road, nobody knew. He would have been safer on the straight, paved road to town.

Before getting to the Turner's ramshackle yard with their two chained watchdogs, I take Barranca down into the wash where the recent waters have brushed the muddy sand in feather patterns. There are a lot of leaves gathered on the stream bed and pools of water. Barranca is unnerved by the sound of the crunching leaves beneath his hooves. Horses seem more easily spooked when they are out alone.

White-boned sycamores and cottonwoods grow all along the way. There is a large field to the left, which the Turners sometimes cultivate with soy beans, and there are many small fruit trees out in the yard. I heard that John Turner's father, Jack, once ordered a large quantity of quince trees, but when they arrived and were planted, they turned out to be pomegranates. It's nice to see the red round fruit still hanging from the grey bare limbs, making holiday for the birds.

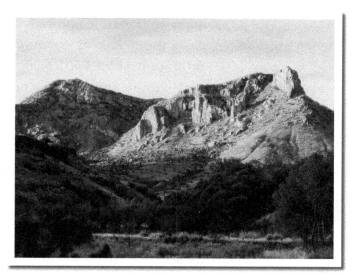

Indianhead Mountain

How I Love to Find a New Trail

Eager to explore the forest road up Indianhead Mountain, I call Sonny McQuiston and ask about the gate with the padlocks. He says that the lock he left there is just dangling from its chain, not really securing anything. In any case, he's fine with me riding up there. I am always grateful when ranchers are lenient.

Phil and Leslie arrive at half-past-ten, and we begin to get all three horses ready, until I notice that Peanut has lost a shoe. We won't be able to take him out. Phil says he can take his dogs hunting and that Leslie and I should go.

We walk the horses for a mile down the road, finding the gate with the padlock. I realize that if I undo the top two wires, I can ease the post out from under the circle of the chain. I put on my gloves so that I won't get cut from the rusty barbed wire, but it's not hard to dismantle the gate—*we're through!*

With a yelp we head up the rolling trail, climbing higher and higher until we are close to the face of the mountain. Quickly, we gain altitude and stop to look back down on the Harshaw Creek Valley with its proliferation of dark--green oaks. As we continue to climb, I spot *Casa Durazno.* Getting out my cell phone, I give Mason a call. "Can you see us? I'll wave my arms." He finds us with his telescope, though he says we seem miniscule against the enormous face of the mountain.

There are many inviting pastures up here that level out as we go. Clearly, this road has not been traveled by truck in quite some time, but we are able to follow the trail and keep wending our way around obstacles. The chartreuse lichen is particularly vibrant on the tall rock face. From this height, we can see all the surrounding mountains covered with snow—*sun on snow,* such a brilliant combination.

On the way down, I spot the old white horse that the Turners have turned out alone on this land. He is so old and wasted he doesn't even move when he sees us. Barranca is interested in what this white horse is all about, but even as we approach him, the horse stands stock still. I worry that perhaps he is not getting enough food and water up here. Horses like to have at least one companion, and this poor old guy is a lonely sight.

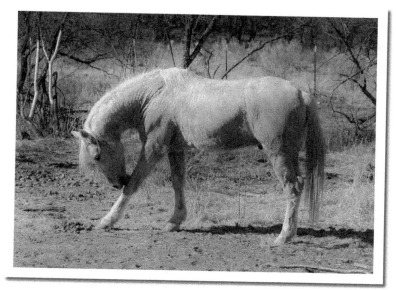

Tonka Waken

Guajolote Flats

I have an afternoon ride planned with Helen but run into Patagonia first to go to the post office. I see Miguel Fuentes, who helps supply our firewood. One time he was helping me clean up the wood pile when a pack rat ran up my sweatpants! We always have a good laugh over *la rata*.

I ask Miguel if he would be willing to do some *trabajo, dos horas, con caballos, ahora,"* and he says, *"Si."* I don't really speak Spanish and he doesn't understand English, but somehow we communicate, I think.

I need help forking up the old, wet hay embedded in the mud around the feeder. But Miguel doesn't show up on time, so perhaps he misunderstood me. Helen and I wait a bit more, then take off for Guajolote (turkey) Flats. The trails here go up high into the Patagonia Mountains. As we climb, we look down on Soldier's Basin where we see a border patrol SUV on a distant red clay road cut into the mountain. We wave. Do they have their binoculars trained on us? I wonder if we look dangerous.

Today, we are seeking out an old mesquite corral that is somewhere up in this direction. Passing through three gates, we finally have the option of bearing right or going down a steep bumpy road to the left. My memory tells me—*left*— and soon we find it. Leading the horses into this broken-down enclosure we think about camping out up here—what fun we would have together.

On family vacations, Helen and I often went riding in the most unusual places, whether it was on the beaches of Mexico or looking for elephants in Kenya. A family trip was not a proper adventure without a horseback ride, and it was a great way for the members of our boisterous, athletic family to be together.

Helen's father, my Uncle Billy, still liked to ride, and owned several Icelandic horses in Vermont, while Popi was in charge of the family stable in Oconomowoc, Wisconsin. It held a motley crew of llamas and Thoroughbreds, purchased off the track, (obviously not winners). There was not one truly sound and steady horse amongst them. People often offered him their rejects, for he never looked a gift horse in the mouth. He did have one or two personal favorites, and Merlin was one of them.

Once when he wanted to give me a piece of jewelry he'd purchased in Tuscany, he took me into the stall of this dappled Arabian, a horse I considered too small for my dad. There around Merlin's neck hung a golden chain with lapis stones. For a moment, I thought he was getting queer for this horse, but no, it was actually a necklace for me.

In the winter Popi rode out in Carefree, Arizona, and he liked to joke that his chestnut gelding had saved his life. On an all-day ride in the desert, my dad had collapsed from heat prostration and had to be collected by helicopter. When they took him to the clinic, the doctors discovered that he was anemic. The anemia led the doctors in Milwaukee to detect esophageal cancer in its earliest stages. Thanks to this riding mishap, a successful operation, and subsequent radiation, he was able to live another six years.

Even after radiation treatment, losing close to eighty pounds, he kept on riding. He rode days before he was taken into intensive care. He rode right up to the pearly gates, I suppose. Don't worry, Dad, we'll take care of Mom and your horses. I wonder where he's riding now.

Helen and I look out over the San Rafael Valley in the distance and feel like we are on top of the world. Few people know the land around here as well as we do, having ridden over so much of this landscape. Today, I feel especially intimate with this great expanse. Our dogs follow nicely, scooting in and out of the red-barked manzanita, which flourishes up at this altitude.

Helen points out the deep grinding hum of a drone somewhere out of sight. These are unmanned glider planes, controlled from Sierra Vista, looking for drug runners and other transients. "Why can't they use mufflers on those things?" Helen protests. We agree that the drone creates an unfortunate noise in this otherwise peaceful terrain. Often we ride in deep silence.

On our way home, every vehicle that passes us on the road is a border patrol van. Three BP men all dressed in green are having a bit of a break by the roadside. Helen stops the truck to chat and asks if there has been much activity in the area. "Yeah, we're always busy," one responds. But they don't look too busy at the moment.

By the time we get back to the corral, Miguel is there working away and I join him. He has already gathered up most of the old rotten hay, and we finish cleaning up together. Most people out West don't bother with manure, letting it dry up and blow away, but we are making compost. I remove three *cholla* plants, which could be potential hazards. Miguel wonders if I'd like a bottle of *bacanora*, tequila moonshine, and it seems like the perfect gift for Clovis when we go to visit him in Australia.

MEXICO

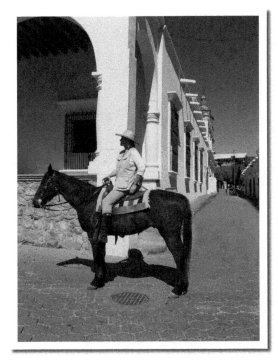

In Town

Off to Alamos

Fifteen months ago, Hurricane Norbert swept over this colonial town dropping twenty-seven inches of rain on the already saturated mountains. Three major mudslides were released, bringing a torrent of muddy water through Alamos, sweeping cars aside, destroying bridges, taking out roads and electricity and leaving the beautiful *Hacienda de los Santos* knee-deep in mud. But even worse, the poor people in the lower land were devastated, often trapped in their adobe homes, holding babies over their heads as the waters mounted.

Now, as Erma Duran and I drive into town, everything looks relatively normal. The lush hillsides of Alamos are covered with the bright magenta blossoms of the *amapa* trees, which are always blooming this time of year when we come down for the annual music festival. It has taken eight hours to get here, and we are eager to unload our bags and settle in.

The next day, my friend Erma goes to work on one of the hacienda's antique wooden statues. Erma has done restoration work all over the world, and she is scheduled to restore the hacienda's little theater with Venetian plaster and stenciling.

That morning, I meet up with an American woman named Linda on the outskirts of town, and follow her pickup to the corral at the end of a twisting maze of unpaved roads. Linda Knieval Damesworth is related to the famous motorcyclist, Evel Knieval, and I wonder if she has some of the same death-defying genes.

I get out my own saddle and pad, as many Mexican saddles have stirrups that are far too short for me, and my Western saddle seems to fit this little mare, Rayulita, perfectly. She is part Arab, and her five-month-old colt is a smart-looking dun, but he will have to stay behind with the other horses as we ride up the cobbled streets on the far side of the wash, waving to the local children who gaze at us from their well-swept yards.

Continuing out into the foothills, Linda points out the *palo santo* trees, which are now bare, a grey-barked tree with white saucer-like flowers that are sweet and succulent. "Hunters often position themselves near these trees because the blossoms draw the animals," she explains.

We jog on down a small dirt road, passing the entrance to *Rancho Palomar*. Linda mentions that many hunters go there to shoot quail and dove, and the chef then cooks them up. The road continues with fragrant, wet sage growing on either side. As we wind up into the higher hills, there is a gradual incline, and I suggest we try a canter.

Rayulita takes off. I can tell she is not used to an easy lope but likes to flat-out run. Her gait is a bit choppy, and I have to hold myself down in the saddle as we leave Linda and her horse behind. At the top of the hill, I wait for her to join us. The air smells fresh—they had quite a bit of winter rainfall the previous week—and I wonder if that will be a problem on our ride over the Alamos Mountains scheduled for the following day.

Big, dark clouds are building, and the lights of Alamos are coming on in the distance. If it rains again tonight, the ride might be called off. Linda thinks that the five-hour ride to *El Promontorio* is a bit arduous—there is a lot of climbing over slick rock and rubble to get to the old mining site.

In 1683, silver mines were discovered here by the Spaniards, and by 1790, mining was at its peak. Alamos produced more silver during this period than any other place in the world. Now new mines are starting back up, which pleases the local Mexicans as that means jobs, a much different attitude than we have in southern Arizona.

On the way back, the sky continues to darken. Rayulita shows me how fast she can walk, eager to get back to her nursing colt. She is a very responsive little mare. I hope I can go out on her again.

I thank Linda and head back into town to join Erma for dinner. Then we race across the street to the opera. Afterward, the crowd spills out onto the cobbled streets where we spot Ramon and his patient white donkey, Gaspar, loaded down with casks of red wine. The young people follow the *estudiantina* singers, decked out in their traditional beribboned costumes. Meandering around the streets of Alamos, the crowd sings along with the instruments, helping themselves to free wine, a very festive tradition.

When we retire for the evening, music still fills the streets from a distance. I want to get a good night's sleep before tomorrow's long ride. I keep hearing warnings about *El Promontorio*, often including the word, *peligrosa* (dangerous), and I'm a little wary as I sit outside in the courtyard and watch the lightning in the Alamos Mountains high above. A light rain begins to fall—good for sleep—but will it make the trails too slippery? While the town is now clean, out celebrating, cat-claw tracks from the recent mudslides are still scarring the mountains as if embedded in natural history.

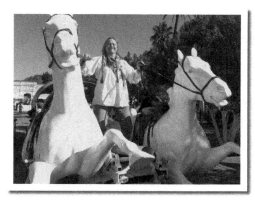

Whoa!

Over the Mountain

This morning is dry and clear, perfect weather for riding, though I have been warned that it could be very cold up in the mountains, especially if we ride into the clouds. I take along multiple layers when we go over to the Red Door for breakfast.

Teri Arnold, the owner of *La Puerta Roja*, has organized our adventure. Another friend of hers, Rosemary Kovatch, will join us. She is a beautiful woman with blonde curly hair and warm eyes, all decked out in a red cowboy shirt and matching boots, ready to go.

But first we feast on the best breakfast in town and have cup after cup of strong coffee. Then Erma heads off to the notary to get the title to her little "ruin," which she purchased three years ago. She will join us for dinner out in Aduana, a small village about fifteen minutes away. Leon, a Mexican cowboy, is waiting for us there with three horses tied to a *chalate* tree, an enormous fig.

Again, I use my own saddle, and Leon admires it, though I have to redo his cinching. I think this annoys him, but I don't want to ride with a large knot of leather under my knee. Leon does not speak English, and despite my blank stare, he assumes I can understand his instructions. I gather that he wants me to keep the horse's head up high as he thinks the horse might trip otherwise, but many Mexican bits are so tough I want to handle her mouth gently.

Teri is all decked out in Argentinean gear—a maroon poncho trimmed in black and a flat-topped gaucho hat. "I might not know how to ride," she laughs, "but at least I look good!"

Leon's nephew is accompanying the ride on foot. They feel they need an extra man along in case anyone gets into trouble. I wonder what kind of trouble they are imagining, but no one thinks that last night's rain will cause a problem. In fact, the earth looks dry. One of the largest fig trees in the area grows near the wash, perched on top of a wall with its rope-like roots streaming down the embankment in a combed out, mud-grey flow.

Quickly climbing up out of Aduana, we comment on the petrified mining sludge that has been left like frozen lava on the hillside. Passing the luxurious home of two renovators, Peter and Bob, we note a flame tree blazing with blossoms in their well-kept courtyard. The long main building was once part of the mining operation, as the mine had to bring silver over the mountain by aerial tram.

There are some stray cattle along the way, accompanied by the sonorous sound of cowbells. The horses know the trail and seem sure-footed. *Pochote* trees (also known as kapok) are scattered here and there. The large seed pods have opened to expose little puffs of white fiber. Sometimes the birds line their nests with this cozy cotton, but the local Indians also gather the fiber, spin it, and use it in their weaving. Long-tailed blue-black magpie jays take off into the mountain air—*exotico*.

Squeezing through one narrow rickety gate, we each take turns ducking under a low-hung tree and scramble up some loose rock to get to the trail. Then it is fairly easy riding. All my fears are blown away. There are no radical drop-offs, only tremendous views.

As we continue climbing, *Casharamba* is dominant in the distance. This flat-topped mountain reminds me of one of Yosemite's majestic peaks. Not surprising that the local Indians consider it a holy mountain. Its name means "needle in the ear" because there is a hole in the base of the rock, like a pierced lobe. I wonder if the wind whistles through there at times, speaking an unknown language to the indigenous.

At the crest, we can see all the way to the Sea of Cortez, and in the other direction—the Sierra Madre and the beginning of the *Barranca del Cobre*, Copper Canyon.

We are headed for the ruins of an old mine that was once owned by the mayor of Alamos. He reasoned that Sonora could use a prison and that the prisoners could help work his operation. This was a prison without bars, because apparently no one had the energy to escape after a long day's work. In fact, the life expectancy of the prisoners after incarceration averaged only eighteen months.

We begin to descend and look out over uninhabited land. It is already getting warm, and we all strip down to our t-shirts, tying extra wraps to the backs of our saddles. After an hour or so, we come upon the abandoned mine buildings, with one towering smokestack made out of well-maintained brick, but the stone foundation of the old hacienda is crumbling. We tie up near another massive fig tree that reminds me of Peter Pan's hideout.

Wandering about the ruins, we come upon a brick tunnel. Walking inside, I smell bat guano and see a mass of tiny bats flying about—disarming. We are told that the prisoners had to enter this tunnel at night, first on their knees and then flat out on their bellies before reaching the sleeping quarters where twenty to thirty men were housed.

Settling down at the base of a fig tree, we share our snacks, though we want to save our appetites for Sam's in Aduana, knowing we'll have a feast of *boltanos*, platters of family-style food. Teri pulls out her cell phone and—guess what—"*No reception!*" Leaning back against the trunk of the tree, we talk about the ride that Teri is going to take with some women-friends in Africa. "I might not be the best rider, but at least I know how to have fun," she laughs.

After an hour's rest, we mount back up and retrace our steps. It is always interesting to experience the landscape in both directions. We can now see the little village down below and the town of Alamos to the west. It is about a nine-mile ride, and as we come into town, we feel triumphant. Cantering up the last stretch of cobblestones toward the church plaza, a herd of goats dances around us. One little guy even bounces up onto the stone wall to get out of our way.

It is only four o'clock and we have an hour before the others arrive for dinner, so Rosemary and I have a cup of tea before we head over to the cooperative shop up the hill. Here local women make all sorts of primitive dolls—the more naïf the better. There are tiny purses fashioned from goats' balls, trimmed in gold with dangling fringe. It is a most curious assortment of finds: tiny, old burro shoes, minerals, hand-stitched pillows, and rustic baskets made from saguaro cactus.

An elderly man takes us into his house at the end of the lane. He has an old carpenter's chest for sale, painted orange and blue—it would make a perfect tack box. When he opens it up, I see that the chest contains all sorts of treasures: a bag of old coins, baby shoes, his passport and other important papers. It seems sad for him to part with it, but he assures me that he wants to sell.

Soon Erma and the others arrive. Sam serves up some excellent margaritas, and we are all ready for the *boltanos* that follow—grilled shrimp, marinated in an orange marmalade mixed with five kinds of chilies, garlic, oil, vinegar, and sugar, delicious, especially because they've been grilled in the shell. We peel and devour them by hand. Then a delectable chipotle-creamed chicken with slices of apple, and another platter of filet mignon and local green beans. Finally, there is chocolate cake and coffee to get us back on the road to town so that we can get to the evening performance. Horses and opera, feasting and fete-ing, all on the night of the full moon.

ARIZONA

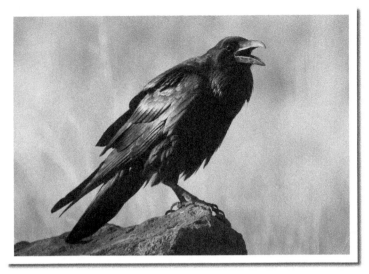

Raven

Part of the Family

Two ravens have made themselves at home in the horse paddock. I assume they have come to gather dropped bits of grain. They sit together on the gate like a pair of old cronies contemplating their domain. I wonder what the horses think of them. Do they consider them part of the herd, part of our extended family?

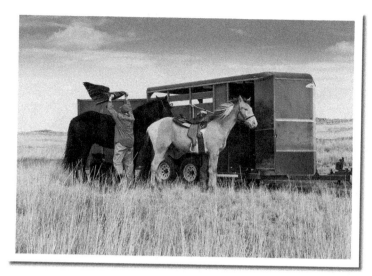

Wind

Definitely an Off Day

Not in a great mood even on waking. *Why.* Is it the wind? I hate the wind as much as the horses do. I even prefer a blizzard or hail to this incessant blowing. They say that the wind carries the scent of predators and that is why horses get spooky.

Helen arrives with her trailer, and then Phil and Leslie show up, but taking all three of my horses out is a lot of work with the machinations of feeding, mucking, catching, grooming, saddling, bridling, and loading. Tonka steps on Phil's foot. Then driving out of the paddock, I ram the side of the trailer into a fence post, bending a fender up against the tire. We have to get out a hammer to pry the metal away from the rubber or we'll have a flat in no time. *Wind.*

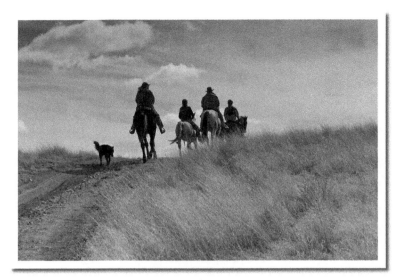

Heading Out

Helen remains calm and patient, even though riding with four people on a day like this seems crazy. Up on the San Rafael the wind is even more intense and the horses are unnerved. Everything seems an extra effort. Phil has trouble with his saddle, slipping, his stirrups too long, uneven, and then he pulls so hard on Peanut's mouth, I have to insist that he ease up. Wind, *wind*, WIND!

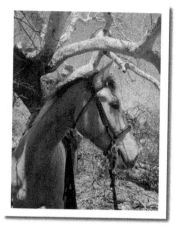

Under the Sycamore

Peanut's Drop-Off Day

Heading to the barn to grain and ready the horses, I groom out all the mud that has accumulated on their coats—little pigpen boys. Barranca gets into the trailer with ease, and then I load Peanut. He doesn't realize that after this morning ride with Leslie, we will be taking him over to Melinda South's for training while I'm in Australia for two weeks.

Mason and I rented a house at the end of Blue Haven Road when we were building our place. I often took long walks with the author Jim Harrison there. He and his wife, Linda, were our closest neighbors. I made their acquaintance by hanging a little bag of New Year's gifts on their gate—a pear, a fire-cracker, and a note asking if it was okay to harvest watercress from the Sonoita Creek that ran by their house. He wrote back immediately, saying, *"NO!" I should not eat the watercress or I might get giardia.* That was the beginning of a good, long friendship, which we have had over these past ten years.

Leslie and I decide to ride all the way to the Harrison's house this morning, passing the Nature Conservancy and then the Circle Z land where I used to ride when I stayed at the ranch with my sons. We cross the creek at the end of the road. The water is deep here, and the horses take a long drink. The Harrison's gate is open so we ride up to the house calling out, "Yoo-hoo, anybody home?" Both Linda and Jim come out to look at the horses. I tell them that we've come for an espresso, and they invite us in. "Just kidding. We've had enough caffeine for one day." Besides, we've got to get back to Melinda's. We're running late.

When we arrive, Melinda's gate is wide open, and her two horses are wandering about the lot freely. Peanut seems a bit nervous eyeing the unfamiliar yard and animals, including a small brown calf named "Steak." We shut Peanut into a pen, get him some hay, and unload grain. I hand over his bridle and attempt to leave a bag of carrots and apples, which could be given to him with his morning feed, but Melinda says that she doesn't like to feed apples because of the carbohydrates. I've never heard that one before. But this is her place, and she is the trainer, so she can call the shots.

Melinda is quite a pistol, a beautiful young woman with long brown hair. She is part Native American, and has a special way with horses.

"I just have one request," I tell her. "Once Peanut is free to roam about the yard with the other horses, can you be sure to close your gate?"

"I'm usually here," she responds, "and I know horses."

But I remain adamant. "I just need you to honor that one request. You know what happened to Helen's horse."

I had given Cody to Helen years ago, and when she came west to build her house in Patagonia, she brought him along. Cody was blind in one eye and thirty-six years old when he escaped his pasture and went careening across Route 82. Spooked, he tried to re-enter his field by crossing a cattle guard where he got his leg stuck and had to be shot, then grotesquely dismembered before receiving a too-shallow grave. It was a terrible end for a truly valiant horse. I had never heard my cousin cry so long and hard as when she received this horrible news.

Melinda agrees to keep the gate shut, but seems a bit put off by my request. Perhaps her horses didn't wander, but Peanut could try to head home. Leaving a beloved horse in someone else's care is a bit like leaving a child at nursery school for the first time. I just want to feel confident and at ease.

"Alpha meets Alpha," I grimace, as we pull on out of the drive.

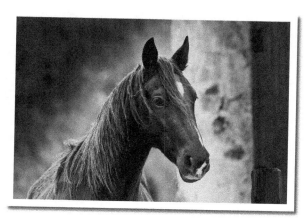

My Best Boy

Grateful

Yet again, I'm entranced by Barranca's beautiful gaits as we ride through the federal land behind the paddock. He is so easy in hand, so willing and wonderful, while Tonka, left alone in the stall, is agitated. I wonder if they both miss Peanut. Do they notice that he is gone? But Peanut is having a fine ole time at winter camp with Melinda South. "He and the filly have fallen in love," Melinda tells me over the phone. Her mean, older, aggressive mare is not quick enough to catch him.

Melinda has more than a few tricks up her sleeve— one is to put sweet feed in a couple of open, lidless, gallon containers, and the horses take turns tossing them about, trying to get out the grain. She also drizzles molasses on some big play balls, and they enjoy licking and kicking the balls. When I drop by for a visit, Peanut comes over to say hello and nuzzles me, then he is off to play with his friends.

Later Melinda calls to tell me that she has gotten Peanut into an excellent flat walk. Her two small sons rode Peanut together bareback, and the older one said, "Peanut is *my* horse."

AUSTRALIA

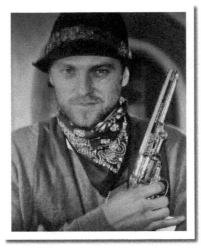

Ayler

A Civilized Ride?

There are over two-hundred horses boarded at the Centennial Parklands Equestrian Centre in Sydney. It is an old-fashioned, well-kept facility that includes five different stables within the complex. A friendly woman recommends Moore Park Stables, so we seek them out and sign up for a ride on March third, which will be right before our flight back to the United States.

I check out their horses and pick Decs for myself. The owner says he is her favorite horse—a strong-looking Appaloosa. Another gelding, Howie, stands 17 hands. Ayler can ride this beautiful bay Thoroughbred. I am just hoping that he won't have an allergic reaction.

The following morning all of us—including my older son, Clovis, his wife and their boys, Kailer and Cash—return to the airport for a flight to Hamilton Island in the Great Barrier Reef. Here we catch a ferry boat to Lindeman Island.

It is wonderful being with my two little grandsons. I only get to see them once or twice a year, and I relish these visits.

Traveling north, we move closer to the equator, and it is sweltering with heat and humidity. The resort is filled with small children who don't seem to notice or mind. Both boys love swimming with their father, and little Cash lights up whenever he sees "Gramma," reminding me of baby Clovis thirty-five years ago.

We have a great day snorkeling out on the reef where fish glide by in an endless variety of forms. My favorite is the curvy purple lip of a giant clam that opens and shuts so languorously. Another day, we take a boat ride to the silica white sand beach of Whitehaven and spend an afternoon in the buoyant sea water. Using Kailer's plastic shovel and pail, I dig out some of the pure soft sand to bring back to my mother-in-law, Em, knowing how she would love putting her hands in it. Later I find out that she tried to eat it!

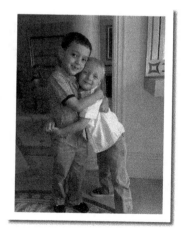

Kailer and Cash

When we return to Sydney for one short night, we rise early for our horseback ride, searching out some good coffee before grabbing a cab for the stable. Unfortunately, my original horse of choice, Decs, is lame. Dante will be his substitute. I decide that Howie is awfully big, and perhaps I should ride him instead of Ayler.

The owner tells us that we will only be able to walk and trot on the equestrian trail that runs around the park. The pathway is separated by a white fence, and the trail itself has good sandy footing. But once we are out, our guide can see that we know what we're doing, and she doesn't mind our cantering on.

There is something so urban about riding in a well-groomed park like this. It reminds me of movies where people are all dressed up in their riding habits, posting in Paris or London or New York—all very civilized, I'm sure, but a far cry from the freedom of the wild, Wild West.

The park must be one of the most beautiful in the world with its undulating grounds filled with plant life and birds, small ponds and playing fields. It is a glorious morning, in the high sixties, refreshing after the intense heat of the Great Barrier Reef. I'm not used to riding on such restricted terrain, but it is still nice to be in the saddle. No trip seems complete without a ride of some sort.

Our guide tells me that Howie is a "bit of a pain," and I soon learn why—for though he has a big strong trot, he is reluctant to get into a canter, and instead of responding to my legs and signals, he simply trots out with bigger and faster strides, until I finally kick him really hard, repeatedly, and then he only canters for a short ways and then drops back into his lazy-boy gait. I might have better luck with a crop, but there aren't even any branches within arm's reach. I have to ride ahead because if she and Ayler canter in front of me, Howie will bolt past them, and I certainly don't want to hurt myself on a strange horse right before takeoff.

Anyway, I am glad that Ayler's horse, Dante, is behaving nicely. We ride by Busby Pond and then the equestrian grounds, where we work the horses in a small ring, but I still have difficulty getting Howie to canter. *What an effort.*

We only have another hour before heading back, so we try to make the best of being out in the fresh warm air. Australia seems especially child-and-dog-friendly. There are strollers and puppies everywhere. One jogging mother goes by at a fast clip pushing her baby ahead of her. The horses seem used to all the distractions and certainly know when they are headed for home. I ask Howie for one final short canter, but when he breaks out of it, I feel a twinge in my back and fear trouble for the long flight home. I will appreciate my own good horses more than ever.

After dismounting, I notice that my inner thigh muscles are stressed, which I have not felt in years. At least I've had a bit of a workout, and Ayler was not bothered at all by the dander. He says repeatedly how happy he is to be riding again. I imagine the day when I can take Kailer and Cash out for a pony ride. What a pleasure that will be.

After showering and packing up, I have to say goodbye to my grandsons. I feel weepy leaving them, not knowing when I will see them again. I have bought each of them a little truck. As they sit at an angle to each other in their highchairs, I kiss them over and over and tell them how much I love them. Clovis ushers me out of the house as I wipe away tears, giving me an understanding hug.

ARIZONA

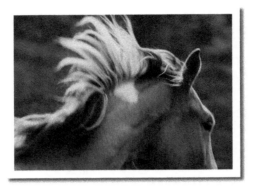

Peanut's Flying Mane

Picking up Peanut

After our two-week trip, we return to Patagonia jet-lagged. When I get up at eight in the morning, there is already a red blinking light signaling a message on my answering machine. I call Melinda back, and she wonders if I can make it over by nine to pick up Peanut before a threatening storm moves in. I thought she was going to have Peanut with her for a few more days, according to our agreement, but I don't want to argue. She considers his training done.

When I arrive, Melinda tells me that Peanut became buddies with the little calf in the next pen. But one night she put the two of them together in the same enclosure—Peanut became defensive of his space and really beat up on the poor little guy. The next morning the calf was all scarred up, shaking, and sorry-looking.

Before I get in the saddle, she shows me some of the stretching exercises she has been doing with Peanut, using bites of carrot to make him turn his head back to touch his side, *treat*, then the other side, *treat*, bending way down, *treat*. I lower her stirrups to the last notch. They still seem short compared to what I'm used to, but she feels that I should have some bend in my knee, rather than riding with my legs hanging straight down.

She is using a halter/bridle combination, which she's willing to lend me until I can get an appropriate bit. Melinda doesn't like Peanut's usual bit that hangs too low in his mouth. He responds much better with a curb chain. She thinks I should buy an Imus Comfort Bit that has a lot of give.

Out on the road, Melinda suggests that I sit back in the saddle more, letting my hips move with the horse, keeping my body relaxed and my shoulders still. This feels right. I get him into a flat walk. He does seem to have made great progress, though it is a bit difficult keeping him going straight ahead.

Then she hops on and works him a while, making him stop and back up whenever he breaks into a pace. This is his reprimand, but when he moves nicely, she releases and praises him profusely. I can tell that he will need a lot of consistency and follow up before this gait locks into his young brain. But Melinda thinks he's a fabulous horse. "He has so much potential, and he hasn't gotten into any rotten habits like a lot of four-year-olds. His fast walk is just like a glide. I really fell in love with him. He only needs to pay attention. Whack him on the rear end if he needs to wake up. There you go."

She admits that she might be getting out of the training business. "It's not the horses, but the people." Was I one of those people? "I'm just not a people person," she confesses. I understand, but we seem to get along pretty well. "It only takes one person to ruin your reputation," she continues, talking about some horse owners that want her to do all the work, but who think they know how the work should be done.

Melinda warns me about letting just anyone ride him. "That could ruin him," she says. "And it's important to warm him up and cool him down with at least fifteen minutes on either end. You can't just cowboy out of the corral." I wouldn't do that anyway.

Back in the yard, we transfer the leftover grain and hay into my truck. Peanut is easy to load. I approach her wild Indian mare, and Melinda says, "She won't let you touch her," but I go ahead and pat her anyway. The mare stands nicely while I stroke her shoulder. Melinda is surprised. Maybe I'm more of an animal person, too.

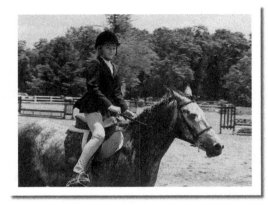

Young Daphne

Daphne's Visit

Nice to have complete trust in one's riding companion, and that is the case with my beautiful, blond niece, Daphne. She has ridden all of her life. One time, when I asked her how high she could jump, she responded, "I can jump just about anything." She began riding with the Fairfax Hunt when she was ten, going at a full gallop for hours, jumping hedges and walls. But when Daphne turned twelve, a friend of her parents fell off during a hunt and was severely injured. Only then did her parents make her stop. She switched gears and went into show jumping, taking fences that were sometimes as high as six feet. I wonder if her parents were aware of this, as they dropped her off at the barn in the morning and picked her up at night.

Getting out of the trailer, Tonka barges by me, knocking me down on the ground. Luckily it is unusually soft earth from all the rains and I'm not hurt, but I realize how I have to practice a more graceful and mannerly exit. I have to assert myself with him so that he knows who's boss.

This morning, we are riding down to the Sonoita Creek near Patagonia Lake. I am eager to see how the water is flowing after all the rain. The long desert slope down to the creek is covered with *ocotillo*. I tell Daphne how the tips of the long cactus wands will soon burst into a blazing red, but it might be another three weeks before the hillsides are painted with that sweep of color.

From this distance, it looks like some of the cottonwoods along the creek have begun to bud out, but we are still a couple of weeks away from high spring. Daphne keeps saying how beautiful it is here—certainly the opposite of New York City, and I am glad that she can give her mind a good airing out. Tonka is going extremely well, especially after we cross the water and head down the well-maintained trail. For the most part, the mesquite branches are at a safe distance from our arms and legs, but I point out some *cholla*, and warn Daphne to give it a wide berth.

I keep to the lead as it makes Tonka more relaxed. I am still having some difficulty with his choppy canter—if he gets in the wrong lead, it really feels scrambled, but if I start him off going up an ascent, he usually goes well, though he will never be as comfortable as Barranca.

We follow the cairns, little towering piles of stacked rocks that mark the way. Moving downstream, we realize that we are the only ones here, not another hiker or rider in sight. It always feels exciting to have this place to ourselves, especially as we enter the area where large bluffs form on either side of the creek—we almost feel like Indian scouts. Finally reaching the long, narrow cave, we tie up both horses, and settle down on the sandy banks of the creek to eat our sandwiches in the sun.

Heading home, Tonka gets into a beautiful fox trot. It's a pleasure to feel him moving forward so nicely. As we climb back up the path toward the trailer, we talk about family. Daphne just spent a couple of nights with my mother in Scottsdale, and Mom's Alzheimer's is getting worse.

Daphne reports that Mom's caregiver, Wanda, described a recent hallucination where Mom thought my brother and I were playing in her fireplace. She kept yelling at Georgie to *Stop It!* He was shaking and choking me and she couldn't get him to quit. This account sends a visceral shiver down through me. Could this be a memory of something that really happened, or was it simply a fabrication of her late-stage dementia?

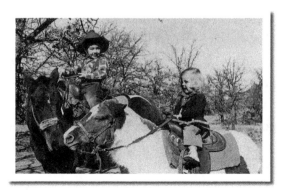

Laura and Georgie

Certainly, growing up, I was not protected from my older brother. The message I received was that it was okay for him to attack me, that no one would look out for me, and that I had better learn how to run. If cries of complaint were taken to our mother-in-collusion, her only response was, "Don't be a tattletale."

But my brother and I were also allies. When my parents were touring Europe, and our housekeeper, Margie, did something twisted, like make us eat raspberries crawling with ants, Georgie would jump up from the table and get on the antique, long-disconnected wall phone and pretend to call the operator, "Help, HELP!" At such moments I applauded him.

If my brother was jealous of me, and cut off my fine, blond hair, trying to make me "be a boy," I do not blame him now, for his behavior was not curtailed. Our mother gave him permission through her neglect.

In retrospect, I think the only one Mom managed to protect from scrutiny was our darling father. She took the fall for him. She became "Mean Margaret," the black hole in our seemingly perfect, extended family, which allowed my father to maintain his pose in his nearly spotless, infallible armor. With her well-used rag, she'd wipe away all telltale signs of his misbehavior and get the dark, oily stain on herself.

For years, every summer, Mom threatened our father with divorce, telling him she would smear his name and misdeeds all over the paper. But then she tried to reason it all away—"This often happens to older men. I wouldn't mind so much if it was with a more attractive person." But of course she felt betrayed. Meanwhile, we all basically turned our heads and blocked her out, immune to her outbursts, unless we were all having dinner upstairs in the carriage house apartment and she rode by on her electric golf cart, stopping down below to announce, "We haven't made love in twelve years! How do you like that?"

I think that if she had been married to a more masculine, dominant man, one who didn't encourage her dark side, she might have been a happier, more loving person. But no one was questioning our father's behavior any more than they were trying to understand hers.

I was the scapegoat, sacrificed on the altar of their misalliance. My presence kept her eyes off of other targets of warranted jealousy. While I knew that he loved our mother and the four of us immeasurably, what he kept locked in the closet of his brain was the most exciting thing!

For some reason it was easy for me to forgive my father. I was more connected to him. When he was recovering from his esophageal cancer operation, Mom left for Arizona, and I was called in to look after him.

When I arrived at Milwaukee's Columbia Hospital, he looked amazingly good, not like death warmed over, as I had expected. His color and humor were excellent. But he was distressed by the tube that ran into his nose and down his throat. He had an IV in his arm, but this nose tube was most disturbing, especially when he tried to talk. But talk he did, for a good two hours, until I realized that I had worn him out. The next day he had a sore throat.

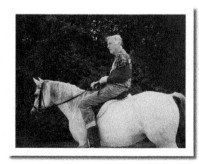

Popi Rides Again

While I was there in the hospital room, Mom called from Scottsdale. It was hard to believe that she had left two days after his cancer surgery. But now I realized that my father had probably urged her to go, knowing that it would make things easier on them both. He was happy to talk to her long distance, and I overheard him telling her that he loved her. This made me feel good, just as it had when I was a little girl and he told me that he loved me very much, but that he loved my mother most. I wished she had believed that.

The last time Reverend Lee showed up at the hospital, Popi told him that he should just pray for him, he didn't need to visit, but here Reverend Lee was again. I found him to be a very likable young man. He seemed particularly open and nonjudgmental.

Popi said he believed that heaven was a spiritual longing common to all people, the idea more important than the fact. "I think heaven is probably on some cloud," he continued, "but I'm not sure which one. I go to Church to support your mother, unless the horses need exercise. Am I damned?"

My father claimed to be an agnostic (not atheist). "I try to follow the teachings of Jesus Christ, but I tend to believe that when a flower dies, its petals are simply blown away—that's the end of it."

The next morning Popi was ready to get that damn tube out of his nose and throat. The nurse had promised him, and he was getting frantic about it. He had held on up to this point and it had tested his patience right up to the end, but now he threatened to pull it out himself if someone didn't come immediately and do it for him. I had rarely seen him so agitated.

I got on the phone, and a nurse rushed in. One simple yank and the deed was done. What a relief. He was so grateful. Popi had not eaten any food for a week, receiving all of his nourishment through the tube that fed into his stomach.

When Reverend Lee arrived, I put a sign on the door—Do Not Disturb—and my father called the nurse's station and said, "No phone calls now. I'm receiving Extreme Unction!"

Reverend Lee read several blessings from the Book of Common Prayer. Then he took some holy oil and marked my father's forehead in the shape of the cross. He opened a silver pyx that he had hanging around his neck. Like a large locket, it opened to reveal the host, a little cross stamped into the middle of each wafer. He put one on my father's tongue and gave me one, too. Then, the three of us held hands and recited the Lord's Prayer. But I heard Popi stop, and I knew he was crying. They say that the Holy Spirit is present when there are heartfelt tears. By the end of the prayer, Popi joined in again, but he was still feeling weak and weepy.

"What do you think Christ meant by: My Father's house has many mansions...I'm going to prepare a place for you?" Then he started to cry again. I stood up and put my hand on his shoulder.

Reverend Lee responded, "I interpret that to mean that God has many rooms for many different kinds of people, space for all. It's my own personal belief that no one will be turned away from God's Love unless he out-and-out rejects God and His gifts."

I believed that no one would be turned away from God's Love, period.

When I told my sister Cia about this, she thought our father might have been concerned about the quality of his residence on the other side—would it be up to snuff? Would there be a mansion on that side, too?

Popi was appreciative of everything I did—the posters I bought to hang on the hospital walls, the egg carton foam pad I got for the bed, the new scrapbook for his get-well cards. It was filling up quickly. I ordered a hospital bed for my parents' apartment, then went out and bought food to stock their kitchen, ordered vitamins, which he would never take, antioxidant tea, which he would never drink, and shark fin powder, which he would return. But mainly, what I did was distract him.

I wanted to do all I could, as if my efforts might make a difference in the final outcome. I wanted to get things set up before my mother came home. I dreaded that changing of the guard, for as much as she said she appreciated what I was doing, I knew underneath that she would be angry at me for doing what she could not.

Finally, the conscience-buzzer went off in her brain, and she realized that maybe she should be in Milwaukee taking care of her critically ill husband. She was suddenly concerned about the cancer that had been detected in his lymph nodes and insisted that he could not get chemo. "Everyone who gets chemo dies."

My weepiness seemed to be an expression of my help-lessness. I found myself sitting at a stop sign, waiting for the light to change until I realized—this was not a light: I could go. I felt as if some part of my brain was displaced, that I could easily forget where I was, where I was going, who I was calling on the telephone. I felt oddly removed, absent from myself.

Then, I braced myself for my mother's return. I had changed her sheets and made her bed. The apartment was immaculate. But on entering the apartment, she started moving bouquets around as if each one had been set down in the wrong place.

She said how wonderful I had been to come and take care of her husband, but then, in the same breath, she went on to tell me how she had played golf on Tuesday and tennis on Wednesday. I was appalled.

"The doctors want Popi to come home on Friday," I told her.

"He's not coming here until Monday when I'm ready for him," she snapped. I guess she needed four days to unpack her things. Wanda was being flown all the way from Arizona to help her rearrange her closet.

The first day home, she had scheduled a hair appointment in Hartland, an hour away, and she wondered if I wanted to go along and have a massage. I declined.

On arriving at the hospital, one of my cousins was visiting with his kids. Mom came in like a fury ordering everyone to leave, insisting that children should not be allowed to visit. He could catch pneumonia. Yes, and he could catch a lot of things spending an extra four days in the hospital.

I could visibly see my father's spirits drop. He was upset by her outburst. He was not strong enough to take it. He told her she should not come to the hospital if she was going to bring so much tension with her. She stayed fifteen minutes, then left. "This is all too much for me."

I suggested that it might be fun to share Chinese takeout with Popi at the hospital that evening, but she wanted to treat me to some new, fancy restaurant, and I felt obliged to go. Once we had settled into our leather booth, she recounted how my niece, Daphne, had gotten so upset about Popi that she started crying at school, unable to finish her exam. Hearing this, I started to cry as well. Mom was horrified. "For heaven's sake, don't cry here in the restaurant!"

I wanted to discuss what the doctors had said and her only response was, "I don't want to talk about him. I'm sick of talking about him."

Everything she said rubbed me wrong—how he could have NO visitors. No phone calls either. Even though the doctors wanted him up, leading a normal life, moving, exercising, getting his metabolism going, but she insisted, "I need some time to rest." As far as she was concerned, he shouldn't have gotten cancer. He shouldn't have done this to her!

On my last day, I brought my father a St. Christopher's medal on a silver stirrup key chain and told him that he would have to take good care of himself. Perhaps, I had been too present, too over-organized, too much in her way, but I felt terrible about the situation as I got ready for departure. I could not see how this transition to home would work for him. I only wished that my sister was there, but she and her family were still in Africa.

When I talked to Mom on the phone from Massachusetts, her anger was palpable. "I wash my hands of him, the whole thing! He's just impossible. I'm not even speaking to him."

One day, I tried for hours to get through, and it was obvious that she had taken the phone off the hook. I wanted to get a release for my father's pathology reports, to have them sent to another doctor who had had success with alternative medicine. When I finally got through around dinnertime, I said to Mom, "You can't just take the phone off the hook for six straight hours. The doctors couldn't even get through."

"Do you have anything more you want to say?" she snarled. "Do you want to speak to your father?" Then, I could hear her yell in the background. "She thinks you are her husband!"

A half-hour later, my mother called Mason crying hysterically and saying that I was such a troublemaker I had ruined their evening, and that I should never call their house again.

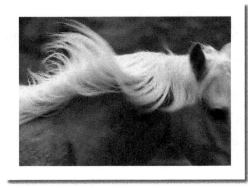

Breeze

Back on the San Rafael

Daphne longs to see the valley, so we decide on a short morning ride, before heading down to Nogales for lunch at *La Roca*. She tries out Tonka this morning, and I take Peanut, who has had several days of rest since coming back from Melinda's. I am eager to see how he will do on the trail now, and he goes beautifully.

It is pleasing to see Daphne's dark silhouette on the top of a rise with all that space surrounding her. She is having a bit of trouble keeping Tonka in his gaited walk as he continually breaks into a canter. She is probably sitting too far forward, and I tell her to let her feet drop from the stirrups as if she were bareback—"That's how you're supposed to sit." At some point, after riding a gaited horse, it just clicks in. One has to listen for the sound of the hooves on the hard-packed road, sounding like "*a piece of meat a shucked potato, a piece of meat a shucked potato...*"

When we do want to go faster, Peanut shows me a lovely little lope that is extremely comfortable. I keep giving him lots of praise as we ride out over the open valley. Leaving the dirt road, we cross the grasslands, toward the headwaters of the Santa Cruz, now filled with water—it is good to see this place transformed back to wetlands from the muddy hole it had been just a month ago.

On the drive home, I take it easy. I have heard that every bump in the road is magnified in the trailer, and that one should drive as if carrying a full tray of champagne flutes. We pass the Hale Ranch where two cowboys are mounting mules. Daphne says how she likes to ride mules when she is at their ranch in Montana, because they are so surefooted and not scared by bears.

One time, when she was only twelve years old, riding out West near Yellowstone National Park at a friend's family place, she went out with five others, up high in the mountains. They were all just standing in a circle when they spotted—"*A bear!*" The other horses all dumped their riders, and some of the people were trampled, but Daphne stayed on. She put herself between the fallen riders and the bear and stared the huge grizzly down until it lumbered off.

Because she was the only one still on her mount, they told her to head back to the ranch to get help. It had taken them hours to get to that point, but she galloped off and came into the ranch house panting. A fancy party was in progress with a lot of New York City and Virginia guests. When she announced that there had been a bear, no one believed her.

They thought she was pulling a prank—at which point, she burst into tears. Only then did they listen to her and send out a helicopter to pick up the injured.

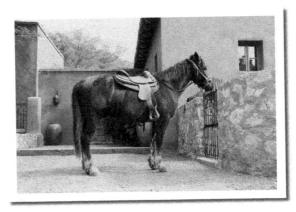

Ready to Ride

Illicit Passage

Helen and I descend to Sonoita Creek, but once we are down, I suggest that we take a right-hand turn on the Cottonwood Loop Trail, which is supposed to be for hikers only, no horses. Helen is game. The two of us have always been apt to break the rules. In any case, we wonder why horses are banned from this trail as there aren't any low-hanging branches. It seems perfectly fine. Perhaps it is a bit wilder here, with a lot of bird life—ducks lifting off from the stream in pairs.

At the far end of the loop, we take another forbidden path up the Blackhawk Trail, until we see a ranger's white truck across the creek, and decide to leave the path and wander upstream through flowing water. Barranca picks his way over the submerged stones. As we proceed up the gradual incline of the river, we turn a corner, and see white water and a forty foot waterfall at the end of the canyon. We are both giddy with excitement.

Riding back up to the edge of the bluff, the footing is precarious, but the horses are only disturbed by one tall barrel cactus that is lying down on its side, rather than standing upright. Helen says one horse she knew was frightened by a felled Christmas tree. Somehow horses know how things are supposed to stand, and their instincts for survival always keep them on the alert, ready to balk or flee. The other day Peanut didn't like the looks of a big brown boulder. Did he think it was a predator or someone in a crouched position?

Passing through the arid desert pasture we come over a rise and are at the same level as Patagonia Lake. There is something so surprising in this that we liken it to the feeling of awe one has driving over the rim of the San Rafael Valley, seeing the abundant grasslands spreading out beyond.

At the level of the spillway, where the water flows from the lake down to the cascading falls and into the creek below, Barranca resists crossing the cement area covered with shallow water, though he has just gracefully picked his way across slippery river rocks and forded deeper water. He must sense that the wet cement could be treacherous.

We decide to go back down into the leafy green comfort of the riverbed, taking the other side of the Cottonwood Loop Trail until it disappears into the unmarked woods. Bush-whacking through the forest on the western side of the river, we make our way back through groves of large mesquite trees, rummaging around. We are not quite sure where we are, but it doesn't seem to matter, other than—*we are not supposed to be here.*

Finally, we find our way back to the trail and then settle down for lunch. I share my sandwich and chocolate with

Helen, as she has not packed anything today. The Saga blue cheese and chicken sandwich with a layer of sun-dried tomato paste is enough to fill us both, and the horses munch. Golden poppies have begun to flower all about their hooves.

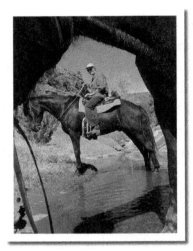

Helen on Ben

Temporal Canyon

I am supposed to meet Helen at her corral at ten in the morning, but at nine-thirty she calls to tell me that Mike is out looking for the horses on their forty-acre spread. After breakfast, Pinto Bean wormed his way out of the corral, followed by Bendajo. The mare, Copper, was so aggravated, she jumped into the huge water trough and out again on the other side to join the geldings. Mike is now trying to round up the horses with his four-wheeler. I suggest that she call me when the horses return.

Later that morning, we head out to Temporal Canyon with Barranca and Ben in tow, winding around through the mountains, the dirt road washboard-rough, but a sweep of poppies has coated the foothills with a profusion of yellow, stunning.

This trail is accompanied by running water all along the way—melting snow from Mount Wrightson, no doubt. It pools in the "blue bathtubs," a place where Helen and friends like to tie up and swim when it's a bit warmer. Today, it is already in the high seventies but not warm enough for a plunge.

The horses enjoy walking through the stream as it crosses the trail, cooling their hooves. The ash trees have just begun to leaf out, looking as if a thousand bright green grasshoppers have alighted on their limbs. Bali lies down in the river every once in a while, perhaps a bit overheated by his growing coat.

Halfway down the trail, something catches my eye—I spot a transient on the far hillside, hiding behind an *agave* cactus as if that spindly plant could protect him from view. I yell out, "*Hola*," but he does not move. We assume that he's on his way toward Tucson, taking this back route through the foothills where he won't be seen by the border patrol.

Wandering on, getting closer to the great peak of Mount Wrightson, we find a nice place to break for lunch. Looking down on the trail, Helen notices a sign spelled out with sticks on the path: "WE HERE." But so are we, and we are ready to eat. I realize I've forgotten to bring Barranca's halter—I'm getting so forgetful these days.

On the way back to the trailer, I keep drinking from my water bottle as the afternoon grows warmer. I suggest that we unsaddle the horses and lead them down to the stream to see if they might like to roll in the nice shallow water, but neither horse wants to do more than take a slurping sip.

After loading Barranca into the trailer, I grab a large plastic bottle from the tack room floor and take a swig—but it is *not* a water bottle—I have just taken a big gulp of floor-cleaning liquid! I spit it out and grab real water and try to flush it out of my mouth, but the toxic taste is hard to get rid of—NASTY. I can feel it burning down my throat.

Luckily, there are no significant repercussions. But when I get home, I sweep out the trailer's tack room, throwing away all the half-empty water bottles and the random junk that has accumulated there. Maybe a little order will help me pay more attention.

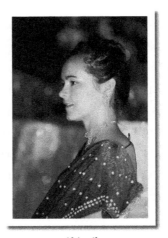

Abigail

Riding with Abigail

After a two-day visit with her grandmother in Scottsdale, my niece, Abigail, is ready to ride with me. Abigail, my sister's oldest daughter, is easy to be with, so calm, she almost floats through the world with her soothing voice. Her relaxed nature makes for a pleasant companion on the trail. I must say that my nieces are faithful granddaughters. Perhaps it is easier being in that generation-skipping role than it is for a daughter like me.

"How's Gramma doing," I ask her.

"Pretty good," she responds. "Thank God she has Wanda." We both agree that Wanda is amazing. Mom couldn't function without her. Wanda is Mom's touchstone, her totally true north, her Rock of Gibraltar, her saving grace.

Abigail goes on to tell me how Wanda was spoon-feeding Gramma lunch, and Gramma almost seemed asleep, her eyes half-closed, but she ate almost all of her soup. "She hasn't been eating much lately. But just as Wanda was getting ready to leave the room, Gramma opened one eye and said, *Isn't there any chocolate ice cream?*"

Abigail grins, and we ride on in silence for a while, but then Abigail adds, "It's so nice that Gramma can be at home. She really loves Arizona."

Mom built her modern fortress of a house years before we built Casa Durazno. She lived in an upper-end, gated community and thought we lived in "no man's land."

At one Thanksgiving in Patagonia, my sister Cia brought her three girls down to our house to join in the festivities. On the car ride from Scottsdale, Mom told Cia, in front of her adopted daughter, Claire, "You know adoption is usually unfortunate, because of the genes."

Claire started crying, "Gramma, you are so mean!"

"I'm never mean," Mom responded.

In contrast, the last thing Popi said to Claire was, "I love you, Claire. I love you as much as all the other grandchildren. Don't ever feel like I love you differently because you are adopted. You are a Chester and that's all there is to it."

Cia took a lot of abuse. Claire was too fat. Abigail had piercings. Lily was rude and unhelpful. I could see Cia wince, receiving this shrapnel. Mom kept talking to Cia about my house, how gorgeous it was, but this compliment came off as a kind of twisted put-down.

Is the pain of rejection so fierce that I now make sure others don't have to feel it? Do I mother my boys with greater love and attention, because of what was withheld from me? Who was I trying to impress with my five-course meals, with my abundant gift-giving? Was it overcompensation or a warped form of spiritual pride?

At least Cia knew how to confront our mother. For some reason, my sister had always been open and direct with her. Cia challenged Mom about how tight she was with her cash—she had some astronomical amount sitting in her checkbook, yet she still quizzed Wanda about the cost of gas and lamb chops. "You know, someday you're going to have to stand up in front of Jesus and explain how you used your money," Cia said.

"If God doesn't like it, that's His problem."

Mom then continued, "Your father was such an idiot, giving so much money to the government." When she tore him down, I tried to switch the subject, derailing her, pointing out the good he had done, putting all of our children through school, but she didn't want to hear about that.

If one of her grandchildren offended her, she would take off like a terror, delivering a scathing litany. It reminded me of all those car rides as a child when I was trapped in the passenger seat, listening to her ongoing monologue. There was never a question of interest in my life, only her ranting opinions. Did she make herself feel better by putting others down? Maybe, it had to do with hormones, or it was just her personality, left unchecked. Certainly, my father never stopped her.

Mom was appalled that Cia's daughters were in blue jeans and t-shirts, not dressed up for Thanksgiving dinner, and that they even brought cans of Coke to the table. I didn't mind, and I was the hostess. I was pleased that everyone liked my delicato squash soup, laced with light cream and Grand Marnier. The turkey was done to perfection. I only wanted to feel grateful that family was together, that we were having a good time and that the sun was shining as only the Arizona sun can shine.

I remember a letter Mom sent me after Mason and I visited my parents in Scottsdale. She was furious because we had decided to go riding with Popi instead of playing tennis with her. If everyone didn't cooperate, she went into a tantrum spreading poisonous fumes over everyone. No wonder we headed for the stable.

"Whose genes are in you?" she wrote to me. "I cannot believe that you are my daughter. You twist your father around your little finger and it is disgusting!"

What can I say? That I don't want to become like my mother, but I am still her daughter. I want to understand what made her the woman she is, but I don't want to replay the inner voice I heard haranguing me since I was an infant. I can still see ticks of resemblance, and notice little facial expressions in photographs, verbal repetitions that are deep in the iceberg of personality formed before I had a choice. But now I do have a choice. And I choose to ride out. I choose to relinquish the past and relish the present, finding freedom and forgiveness on horseback.

Helen is going to meet us at the Patagonia Lake corral at ten. I am riding Tonka, as he seems to do well on this trail, and Abigail has Barranca. On the way down the slope we note new signs of spring —pale mauve bottle-brush flowers and some Indian paintbrush, as well as little purple star-shaped flowers, lovely. The cottonwoods are almost fully leafed out now, and the day is warm and brilliant. There is nothing more beautiful than desert sunshine filtering through those bright spring leaves while riding through creek water. We forge the stream every chance we get and ride for long stretches through the shallows. Tonka is a bit hesitant when he sees long strands of green slime streaming beneath him, but soon he discovers that this is not to be feared. In fact, it might even be edible.

Abigail is enjoying herself, splashing along. We take a few fast gallops along the straight paths, and at one point, Tonka bucks and veers, and I feel a twinge in my spine. He doesn't like to be last, but he's got to learn to behave.

We ride all the way to the gate that leads to Rio Rico. It is as far as we have ever gone, and Helen feels it is far enough. We wander back up through the stream, cliff swallows wheeling overhead, until we find a good place to tie up the horses in the shade. Taking off our boots and socks, stripping down to our underwear, we cross back over into the sun and eat our lunch. A half-hour later, it is not so easy getting sandy, wet feet back into socks and boots. I can feel little pebbles in my pants as we remount, but this lazy break was worth it.

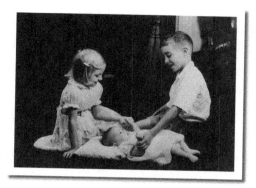

In Front of the Fire

Easter Sunrise

Abigail and I decide to get up at 5:15 A.M. to go for an early ride. After a double espresso, we load up and head to the San Rafael Valley. The morning light is just beginning, and by the time we arrive at the rim of the valley, it is getting brighter. The sun is supposed to rise by 6:08 A.M., though it takes a few extra minutes for it to climb above the Huachucas. The folds of the foothills make a spectacular vision—the lower hills appear darker, scattered with oaks, and a misty lavender haze washes over the paler mountain range behind.

I decide to take Ab to the north end of the valley, and along the way we spot a dead coyote on the road, probably shot by some rancher. Now it just lies there, decaying, but it still has a lovely, intact tail. We ride all the way out to the edge of the valley where I spot a dirt road that seems to be going up the backside of Saddle Mountain. I have often tried to find a way through the fence out here in the hopes of climbing this incline, never meeting with success. But today we find an unlatched gate—*an Easter opening!* We continue to climb until the trail becomes very steep. We have to stop and let the horses rest along the way. I wonder who would make a road up here and for what purpose? Phil Caputo once told me that drug smugglers used the top of Saddle Mountain as a lookout post. Were we riding into danger?

We inevitably talk about Abigail's mother, my sister Cynthia (Cia), five years younger. I loved my serious, little sister, who wrote haiku and absentmindedly walked into trees while contemplating some grand philosophical thought. True, I had been jealous of my father's taunting, saying over and over—"Cynthia has the most beautiful hair in the family." Her luscious auburn locks were the same color as my father's when he was a boy. My darling dumpling of a sister was not a serious threat, but his terrible teasing drove me (a straggly haired blonde) to snap off forsythia wands and whip them against various objects. This is For-Cynthia, and this!

I can remember how mortified I was when my mother exclaimed, "You're just jealous of your sister."

"No, I'm not," I lied.

My father used jealousy as a clever tool, a major psychological weapon in his arsenal. He used it to protect himself. He used it as a smokescreen, setting us up like figurines, moving us into position, so that we would be jealous of each other, instead of focusing on his faults. But I was tired of being pitted against mother and sister, for what? So he could have his illicit freedom—running off to Paris or San Francisco for some dangerous fun?

For a long time our family dynamic had been distorted, and no one had been honest about the source. All anyone ever did was complain about Mom, and finally, I had to ask myself—why was she so hostile and angry? I think my father had to take some responsibility there.

I wasn't standing in judgment of him. I knew he preferred a life of fun and games, sneaking around. I could sympathize with what he had had to juggle throughout his life, but when secret desires and needs for escape dominated reason, when naughtiness and rebellion against the maternal were continually acted out, there could not be a clear sense of boundaries, where the adult cares for and protects the child.

Of course, I am only realizing this now, as a woman and a mother. As a girl I just went along with whatever unsettling schemes my father had. Throughout my childhood, I never asked, "Is this normal? Is this parenting what others experience?" Only the adult-child in remembrance tries to put the pieces together.

I remember when Geoff, my first husband, and I were having a difficult time in our marriage, my father offered to send us to Door County for the weekend, while he took our three-year-old Clovis to the Wisconsin Dells. We agreed, and had a terrible time. When Clovis returned from his outing, he ran wildly into my arms. I looked up at my father wondering—what's wrong? "What happened?"

"Popi threw me into the pool," Clovis said.

"He doesn't even know how to swim!"

My father looked sheepish, but I was aghast.

And why did my father want to terrify me in the waves of the Atlantic when I was a small girl? He put me up on his shoulders and went out deep—the salty water going up my nose, making me gag. I have been a coward in the surf ever since.

When I was eight, my father put me on a city bus in downtown Milwaukee and told me to get off at the Downer Avenue stop, our neighborhood. This ride must have taken a full half-hour or more, and all along the way, I felt displaced and anxious, wondering if I would get lost. Would I recognize the popcorn stand, the bike store across from St. Mark's Episcopal? Once I got home, I was rattled, as if I'd been put in harm's way.

Many years later, I heard my sister's story. She and our younger brother, David, were having their childhood European tour with our parents, and while in Venice, my father let go of her small hand in the middle of the Grand Piazza. He told her to stand there, alone, and he would watch from a distance. He wanted to see who might try to pick her up. Cia went along with the game, uneasy, yet acquiescent.

I remember how he left my twelve-year-old brother, Georgie, in the middle of Dublin, all alone in a large strange city, because he was lagging behind. I was alarmed that he would abandon my brother, and was probably even more upset than he was. Luckily Georgie had a book of matches in his pocket with the name of our hotel.

And why would my father want to subject me, a lithe, attractive teenage girl, to a dinner with a well-known sex offender? David Tallmadge was a Schlitz beer heir and my father's client. The three of us sat together at the Oconomowoc Lake Club, and during the whole meal, Mr. Tallmadge leered at me from across the table. I had never experienced this kind of lasciviousness, and it made me extremely uncomfortable.

Cia and I agreed that we were not well-protected as girls, and perhaps we were overreacting as adults, but maybe that is the see-saw of generations: Much passes from one to the next, like a ledger book, until someone finally does some accounting.

It's not as if our father was a tough guy, but perhaps because he was the opposite of tough, he wanted to harden us up, so we wouldn't end up being sissies. Was he afraid of appearing to be one?

As a child, I was comfortable being father-identified, claiming I wanted to be a cowboy, never a cowgirl. I always took the male part during my all-girls' school square dances, dressing up in blue jeans and handkerchief scarf. I only put on girls' clothes for Sunday school, holidays, and Christmas cards, where I might be seen playing with my baby sister on the Oriental carpet before a roaring fire. I didn't feel like myself in crinoline, and there was little nurturing of my femininity. My mother was not eager to doll me up. Dresses felt unfamiliar, wrong. I was eager to get out of them as fast as possible, comfortable in my brother's hand-me-downs. I was even put into his swimming trunks, while my cousin, Helen, one year younger, wore a frilly, girlish one-piece.

No childhood is ever perfect. But in retrospect, I am still grateful for the smell and taste and feel of mine. Despite the cruel teasing and horrible pranks, I enjoyed most of our boisterous family fun. I wasn't a sissy. I was a tomboy. But a tough exterior can hide a sad vulnerability beneath.

Sometimes I felt like I was looking back at my genetic stream under an archaic microscope, seeing at last, the source of my gifts and my failings, little signposts, forgotten memories, stumbling blocks, egg on shirt, spills, and stains, unburied treasure.

I had always been a "daddy's girl," but deep down, I wanted to win the heart of my mother. I'd pull up lilies of the valley from their sucking stems to make a fragrant handful for her. I'd write her a poem or make her a picture. I was always trying to please her.

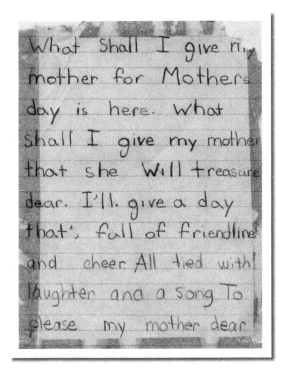

What Shall I give my
mother for Mothers
day is here. What
Shall I give my mother
that she Will treasure
dear. I'll give a day
that's full of friendliness
and cheer. All tied with
laughter and a song To
please my mother dear

Abigail and I clamber over a loose rubble of rock and keep
going until the road runs out. Down below, we can see the
rooftops of the Blackwell Ranch, as well as the pink octagonal
home of our closest neighbors, and there in the distance, the
tiny town of Patagonia. I feel exhilarated, especially nice to take
this ride with my beloved niece early on Easter morning.

We return home to rest up for our midday feast at the Hard
Luck Ranch, home of Gayle and Bob Bergier. Jim Harrison
has his writing studio up at their place off the Salero Road,
and we have all shared this Easter meal together for years—a
fine repast of smoked Virginia ham, German potato salad and
Gayle's exceptional coleslaw with sliced peppers and jicama.
Gayle is also an exceptional baker. Her cupcakes with a light
lemony buttercream are the icing on the end of a great visit
with Abigail.

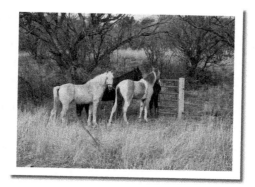

At the Gate

Hog Heaven

Finally, a calm day and I am off to ride with Peter Phinney in Hog Canyon. When I arrive, Peter is already riding Wesley out in the working arena, which has nice soft footing with a clay base. I unload and saddle up Barranca, but when I come around the side of the barn, Peter's horse spooks and spins, throwing a shoe. Does this mean we will have to cancel? Peter goes looking for his tools and manages to pull out the remaining nails in Wesley's rear hoof. He thinks that if we stay on the dirt, we can still have a short ride. So we head down this little wind-protected valley full of dense oak trees. The oaks, which lose their leaves in the spring, are now turning a russet-golden color in preparation for their false fall. The old brittle leaves can leave quite a mess, but I must say that it is nice to have their greenery all winter long and to see the fresh soft leaves appear in early spring like cut velvet.

A large trough by the second gate has a handy little in-and-out ramp for any animal that might get trapped in the water. Peter's two dogs run up it and have a drink but Barranca is wary of the huge slimy tub. Back East, I put a long branch in my water tank so that squirrels and chipmunks can rescue themselves. There is nothing more disturbing than finding a dead, bloated animal tainting your horse's water supply.

Peter is especially happy that I have come out to ride with him as it gives him a chance to make his gelding pay attention to him rather than to another horse. Peter likes the looks of Barranca and how he moves, but because of Wesley's lost shoe, we don't ride up on the ridge or go too far. Instead, we head back to do some flatwork in the ring. I push Barranca into figure eights, cantering him slowly, while Peter practices spinning his horse.

In the show arena, reining horses are spun around four times in each direction. They also have to know how to do a sliding stop, and some horses can slide for almost twenty feet. "It's kind of silly," he admits, "because there is no real need for a sliding stop. It's all for show. And each year, there is some new horse that can go even further."

Peter offers to let me use his wash stall, and it is warm and cozy from the heat lamps above. He even has access to hot water and a nice spray hose that you can adjust. We cross-tie Barranca and wet him down before applying shampoo with a sponge. Then I rinse him thoroughly, mane and tail and all. Scraping off the excess water before using the shedding tool, I get a lot of his loose winter coat off until it looks sleek and shiny. Peter sprays Barranca's tail with a generous amount of a detangling product, and I work on the long strands. There is something satisfying about cleaning a horse—it makes the inside of a woman feel good.

I ask if we can measure Barranca, as I want to know if he is actually 15.3 hands, or possibly taller. Measuring to the middle of his withers, it seems clear that he is a good 16 hands. My Big Boy. We leave him tied to the fence to dry while Peter shows me his Turnbow trailer. It must be the most elegant trailer I've ever seen, deluxe. It has a side ramp, which allows a horse to enter with his head toward the rear. If given a choice, a horse will usually stand with his head going toward the back rather than toward the front, as most trailers are designed. I wonder why horses would prefer riding backward. Maybe they are trying to avoid the wind of the road. Horses always seem to turn their rumps to an approaching storm, perhaps for the same reason.

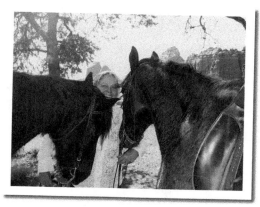

In Sedona

Ready to Roll

So much planning for our trip to Sedona—Helen and I load up the night before—measuring grain into baggies, stashing hay in the back of the truck, getting all of our tack into the trailer, both coolers, not to mention our suitcases, as well as my humidifier and espresso maker! We want to have an easy and smooth departure the next morning. Kathleen

James, our friend, will drive her own car up to Sedona and meet us there for dinner.

We eat sandwiches along the way and only stop once near Picacho Peak to fill up the truck and give the horses slices of apple to moisten their mouths. Climbing out of the congested Phoenix traffic, we leave Highway 10 and enter a barren high plateau that reminds us both of Scotland.

Helen amuses me with tales from her childhood. How her parents would dock five cents from her twenty-five-cent allowance if she said the word *Gol* (too close to God) or *shoot* (too close to shit). We talk about our grandmother, Alice, mother to both of our fathers. Helen says Gramma's funeral was more green than black because there were so many Girl Scouts present. Helen's memories are always different than mine. I think I was grieving too much over the loss of my grandmother to notice what anybody was wearing.

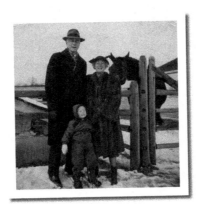

Papa, Gramma, Laura

Soon we see Sedona's red rock mountains in the distance. I had forgotten how grand and awesome this area is. As we pass through Cave Creek, we find the turn off for Jack's Canyon Road, and then the final righthand turn into Horse Mesa Ranch—a lovely boarding situation for our two boys. I think they feel like they are at summer camp, happy to settle into their adjoining stalls with fresh hay and water.

The owner of the facility is there to greet us. The place has a relaxed atmosphere, with about fifty or more horses in regular boarding. Dogs and mules roam about the lot. We uncouple the trailer from the truck, leaving our horses in their open-air stalls. It feels light and free traveling the next stretch without a load behind us.

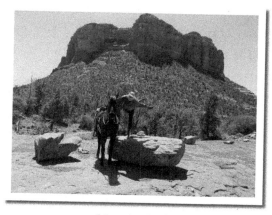

Mounting Rock

My Birthday Ride

Helen, Kathleen, and I are all staying in Mom's comfortable two-bedroom casita at the Enchantment Resort outside of Sedona. Her place is currently up for sale since she never uses it anymore. It is a wonderful spot, far from the tourist shops, with winding trails beneath the dramatic cliffs and hoodoos where "vortex" energy supposedly exists.

Today is the thirteenth of April, my birthday. Fresh orange juice has been delivered to our door in a little wicker purse.

I make eggs with green chile, and we have a leisurely breakfast out on the deck. The red cliffs are just across the way, and the air smells full of fresh pine.

Back at Horse Mesa Ranch, our big boys are waiting for us. Once saddled, Barranca seems especially excited this morning. He dances around while we wait for our guide to get ready—then we follow her down the drive, passing through the surrounding suburbs until we find the gate that leads us out toward Bell Rock. Here we thank our guide and say goodbye. She has filled our heads with so much information about various trails that we have not been paying much attention to the route. We figure we can just follow the paths and pick our way back.

Heading out over a flat plain, we take various turns on red earth that is luxuriously soft after the hard-packed trails of Patagonia. It is a perfect riding day with bright blue sky, warm but not too hot. We canter along these flat, comfortable paths, passing hikers and mountain bikers—a lot of people out enjoying the scenery in this glorious terrain. Bell Rock does indeed look like a big earthen bell, or maybe a teapot without spout or handle. At first, the horses seem a bit unnerved by all the foot traffic, but soon they settle down and are good company for each other, as are we. I feel lucky to have my closest cousin as a regular riding companion.

Helen always came through for me, remembering my birthday and Christmas, traveling across country to attend my father's memorial.

We almost didn't have a service because Mom insisted that there would be none. She didn't want to come back to Milwaukee. Scheduled for knee replacement surgery, she didn't feel up to the trip, even though her doctor had told her that she should be up and walking, leading a normal life.

The four of us siblings had a conference call and decided that we had to have a proper funeral for our father. He had been too important to the community, and our extended family needed a time to come together and grieve. "Closure" was not really the point. For some, there would never be closure.

Together, we decided to override our mother's wishes. When we told her of our decision, she went ballistic. How dare we go against her! I urged her to join us. Mason and I could take her to the airport and fly with her. It didn't seem right that she would boycott her husband's funeral. We would have to make excuses for her, as usual.

But her decision, oddly, felt normal. Popi might have even appreciated her egocentric ways, for it confirmed what everyone thought—that she was impossible and that he was a saint for putting up with her. It was quite a role she had served as his foil. People rarely suspected him of being anything other than a cross between a perfect prince and the good-time guy who always picked up the bill.

The funeral was held on a sunny, balmy mid-March day, and most of our family was present. The mild-mannered Broadoaks caretaker (labeled by Mom as "a moron") had managed to bring a well-groomed llama and horse by trailer from Oconomowoc into Milwaukee. The animals stood outside the front door of the church with leis of flowers around their necks. True Popi style!

My brother, David's, eulogy was a highpoint: "Dad was a joiner who relished the dynamics of the group. He was a habitual includer (never an excluder), and his motto whenever asked if one more person could come out for the weekend was always

*immediate and predictable—'The more the merrier!' He cut
a swath through the world and had enormous fun doing it."*

*Abigail, my niece, also took a turn. "When we were little,"
she began, "my grandfather would on occasion turn into a polar
bear. He would get down on all fours, roaring, and chase
us around the house. For my grandfather, every moment was
a potential adventure, every stranger a potential friend. He may
have been a respectable lawyer and investor in the eyes of the
community, but to his grandchildren, he was a hero."*

*Two weeks after our father's funeral, Mom was going through
her own private season from hell. She went in for double knee-re-
placement surgery. I think it came as a relief to exchange her
emotional pain for physical suffering.*

*I came up to Scottsdale numerous times during her recovery.
Once banished by my mother, she now encouraged me to come,
as if it were the most natural thing.*

Clambering over rock, picking one path or another as the
trail splits, we find ourselves on the less inhabited Llama
Trail, which makes me think of my father, who raised llamas
in Oconomowoc. People always stopped by the field to ask,
"What are they?" *Llamas.* "What are they like?" *Gentle,
alert, prancy.* How he would have enjoyed riding here in the
Munds Mountain Wilderness. We feel at ease picking our way
as we ride along with no concern about how we will return.

My cousin points out grey-blue juniper berries that have
fallen on the red earth with little pokes of fresh grass finishing
the picture. There are lots of one-seed junipers with leaves
called scales instead of needles, pinion pine, and manzanita,
which have a sensually smooth, red-brown bark. The winter

rains have brought out a scattering of wildflowers—purple dick, Indian paintbrush, and little yellow daisies.

The horses drink from the shallow water of the rock pools, slurping it up between their teeth. We choose a high, flat area to tie them up for lunch. In the middle of this open space, there is one large rock where Helen dismounts. The horses are used to getting a treat at their rest stops, and I have a couple of carrots and nibbles in my saddle pack. Loosening their girths, we tie them up in what has to pass for a bit of shade, then we settle down for a rest.

Ready to ride again after lunch, Helen scrambles back up onto the "mounting rock." She is always adept at finding a place to get back onto her tall black horse. Heading down the trail, we choose to go around Courthouse Butte. This loop trail is much wilder with fewer hikers, bikes prohibited, but horses seem to be allowed everywhere.

Our boys do well on the rougher trails, always choosing the best footing, and from time to time, I stop to use the little camera Mason gave me for my birthday, documenting this amazing terrain. The Canon camera flattens out to the size of a pack of playing cards and fits easily into the snap pocket of my shirt.

As we circle around to the front of Courthouse Butte, I insist that our return path is further west. We are back on soft footing, and we get to canter some more, but at a certain point, Bendajo stands stock still and refuses to follow, as if he has had enough for one day and knows we are not headed home. "It's this way, I'm sure," I call back to Helen, but her horse will not budge, so I turn and follow them, and sure enough, Bendajo takes us back to the exit gate. A horse's sense of direction is not to be second-guessed!

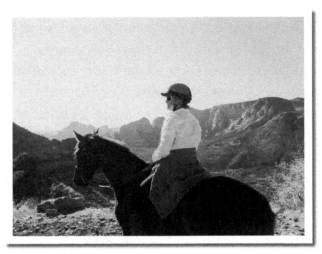

On Top of the World

Helen's Day

Ready for our afternoon ride up Schnebly Hill, a short trailer drive from the stable, we choose the first parking lot we see, hoping we will find the equestrian path.

Finally, we see a sign and drop down to a little pool to let the horses drink, not noticing that the trail continues on the other side of the stream. It isn't until we see an immense, round-shaped rock with a large wide skirt of land around it that we finally connect to the trail. Here we look down on several huge pancake formations that could be UFO landing pads, petrified batter that has flattened out and hardened over time.

Up on the rim of this round mountain we take a break and look back down the valley. I give the horses a couple of Tic-Tacs, and they nod in approval. Up higher, we can see how the road climbs, and decide on making it to a high lookout point before returning back down the mountain. The afternoon sun is warm, and I tie my jacket around my waist. It takes us another half-hour to climb up to the lookout but it is worth it—we can see such a distance it makes us feel small, a small part of this extensive grandeur.

Helen understood my history, my struggle with my mother. She would often sigh, a deep heart-felt sigh, but she rarely made a negative comment. While I was growing up, my mother had been the target of endless jokes, which were hurtful to me as a girl. No matter how much I suffered under the rule of "Mean Margaret," a child can only be defensive in the face of such put-downs.

No one ever pointed a finger at Popi, for he was part of the dynasty. He was the fun one, the life of the party, the upbeat one. No wonder he was on so many executive boards. He made those old men laugh, leading his llamas into various meetings, arriving in costume, planning a prank or pulling a gag.

But now it seemed as if the family dump site was being excavated by Mom's grief. She was just a sore, scraped plot of turf. And it was time for me to plant some growing things, time to find forgiveness. I kept trying to locate my storehouse of sympathy. I realized that being a target, she had needed her own victim.

I fit the role, being the favored, oldest daughter. I took Dad off to the country to ride when she wanted him at home in River Hills. She was insatiable for his company, and struck out at anyone who challenged her claim.

After a horseback ride, I was asked to pull off my father's big black boots, tugging at the close-fitting two-toned leather. I remember the smell of man musk on his feet and horse-fresh dander on his thick beige jodhpurs. Was this innocent contact too intimate for her?

But now she was just an old woman who could not stop crying. She was furious with him, for many reasons. She ranted and raved, but bottom line, she missed him terribly. She was lost without him. For the first time in her life, she was alone and missed him like a lake sucked dry. She was trapped in a nightmare with dull dark dread. No teasing, no conversation at the dinner table, no bantering before the TV, no backdrop, no husband.

Instead of giving up chocolate or caffeine or wine for Lent, I decided to call my mother daily. I no longer cowered around her. On the contrary, I told her what to do and got a little bossy, but she was flattered by the firm and consistent attention. "You need to find a physical therapist," I insisted. "You should be getting a weekly massage, and at least one pedicure a month."

Returning home from her operation, my mother's brother came for a visit, driving all the way from Augusta, Georgia. He was an excellent chef and cooked elaborate meals every night. When I called, it sounded as if they were having an almost manic, hilarious time, but hours after his departure, in a state of careless exhaustion, my mother slipped on the carpet by her bed, fell down, and broke her hip.

Two weeks out of the hospital, she now had to return for hip replacement surgery. More pain, more tears, more angst. This operation was harder to take. She didn't have her pick of doctors. She didn't have the same good rehab facility. Would there be no end to her suffering?

Coming back down the mountain on our horses, we decide to follow the trail all the way to the bottom. It is a splendid little path that winds down beside the running creek. At one point, we come through a wonderland of cactus. It looks like it could be a botanical garden, wildflowers scattered all along the way.

Back at Horse Mesa Ranch, some new arrivals, Buzz and Cathy, have just pulled in from Pennsylvania. They offer us gin and tonics, so we sit down outside their large house/horse trailer and put up our feet, drinking and talking until the sun goes down.

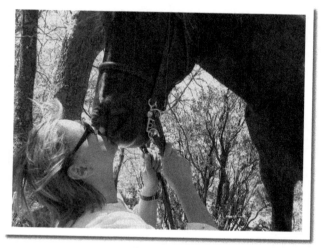

Connected

Brisk Barranca

We woke to snow yesterday morning, snow, at the end of April. But today, everything has melted, and it is brisk and moist. A Mexican Jay flits about in the mesquite, and the air is as cool as fresh cucumber. I have such a heart connection with Barranca and just hope that he will go on and on, healthy and happy. He is always so willing, as if he wants to please me. How lucky I am to have found this horse, my perfect equine companion.

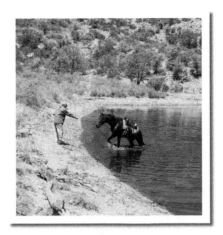

All Wet

Cochise Stronghold

As we drive toward Dragoon, Helen reads from the tear sheet Mason has printed off the Internet: *Cochise Stronghold is a protective rampart of granite domes and sheer cliffs that was once the base of operations for famed Chiricahua Apache Chief, Cochise. Sentinels, constantly on watch from the towering pinnacles of rock, could spot their enemies in the valley below and sweep down without warning....Upon his death, Cochise was secretly buried somewhere near his impregnable fortress. The exact location has never been revealed.*

Turning toward the mountains the road becomes dirt, rippled with washboard ridges. The equestrian parking lot is just a half-mile up ahead next to an old, abandoned, stone house. When we pull in, we see that we are the only riders in the stronghold this morning—*nice.*

Heading down the trail, we meet three middle-aged women on foot with their tiny dogs. They suggest that we take the Middlemarch Trail instead of the Cochise Trail, which is difficult for horses to traverse with its narrow cuts and switchbacks. I say, "Thanks," but I should have said, "*No thanks,*" as the Middlemarch Trail turns out to be extremely rocky and uninteresting with low cedar growth and no significant vistas. We keep on climbing for about an hour, going through three gates before we get to a rise and see more of the same ahead.

"What do you think?" I ask Helen. "Maybe, we should turn back and try the other trail." I remember it as being spectacular, and this is rather boring. She agrees, so down we go. In the distance, we spot a large watering hole, and decide to stop and have our lunch here before riding up the Cochise Trail with its grand domes of stacked rock.

Helen lets Bendajo wander around untied with his hackamore knotted over his pommel. But then he takes it upon himself to wade out into the dark water up to his belly. He is about to submerge, saddle and all, when Helen gets him to return. I hold onto Barranca's reins, and he stands over me, looking for treats, grabbing mouthfuls of grass where he can. I realize how much I trust this horse and feel a rush of affection for him.

After lunch, we find the turnoff for the Cochise Trail and are immediately entranced. The path winds around through alligator juniper, century plants, and prickly pear cactus, affording constant views of the unusual mountains that look like balanced piles of smooth stone stacked up by a giant three-year-old. We have to pass over one difficult, slick section, and the horses pick their way down a steep staircase of rough rocks, but they both manage, sure-footed. I only wish that we had time to ride all the way to the top.

We imagine all the hiding places that Cochise and his tribe secured. The leader's wild spirit seems to float over this landscape as if inhabiting the repeated call of a mourning dove. I answer—calling back—pretending to be an Apache speaking in native code. When I bring up our grandmother, Helen says, "I was just thinking of her!" Maybe, her spirit is hovering about us, pleased that her two oldest grand-daughters are exploring these wild mountains together.

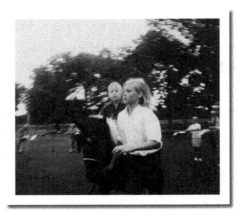

Homestyle Horseshow

Helen and I were always getting into trouble as adolescents, going out into the horse field to sneak a smoke behind the jumping log, or riding bareback in the moonlight, only to discover that our horses had escaped their pasture after our wild midnight ride.

Our grandmother was a very moral, upright person. She disdained TV and called it, "Truck." She never drank or smoked or even chewed gum. She was horrified when I came home from a summer in France and had started drinking coffee. She repri-manded my mother, saying, "But that is caffeine!" My mother's response to that was—"So what."

Gramma and my mother were impossibly different. My mother was southern, glamorous, passionate, yet poor. Unfortunately, these two women were thrown together in such close proximity that it must have been very difficult for them both. But perhaps their differences were what had attracted my father to my mother in the first place, after his highly-supervised, insulated upbringing.

My grandmother nearly insisted that my mother convert to the Episcopal Church when she married into the family. Early on, Mom's heritage was questioned. My Aunt Isabelle wrote a letter questioning my mother's genes—how important genetics were to a family, and how my father's fiancée was one of the "Chosen People." Certain negative traits might be passed down through the blood, my aunt wrote, as if my mother's background would be a stain on the purity of the family.

Curiously, there seemed to be even more fuss over my mother having been raised a Catholic. My grandmother was very concerned about how this would affect my father's marriage and the raising of his children. She wrote to him at length— galled by the thought of ignorant, superstitious priests telling children a lot of poppycock. "It seems terrible to tell as Gospel truth to credulous trusting little minds, things which you cannot accept as intelligent concepts."

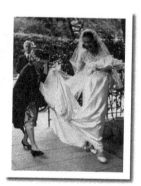

Wedding Day

Mom was convinced that being an Episcopalian was not much different from being a Catholic, but she kept the Jewish part of her history hidden. In Germanic Milwaukee, one couldn't even join the country club if you were part Jewish.

My grandmother took me under her wing and became a significant maternal figure. Strangely, Mason's mother,

Em, reminded me a great deal of my father's mother. Perhaps, that's why I became so close to her. When you can't get along with the parent you've been given, it's natural to choose a loving substitute.

Why are families so important? It's as if we are dealt a handful of cards and we simply have to play them, or close. We can't select our brothers or sisters or parents, though some think the unborn do choose, a charming notion. I can see how I might have picked Popi, but I have to dig deeper to uncover the reasons for selecting my mother. Maybe, she was part of the package deal, or she was my daughter in some past life, and I had not been very nice to her. Was this my chance to get it right?

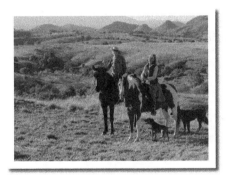

Cowgirls

A Watched Moon

Helen and Anita arrive on the rim of the valley right after I do, Anita wearing one of her fabulous, quirky outfits, blue jeans under her splashy pink and yellow dress, with a beaded, blue cashmere sweater and sparkly glasses. She is always a soothing balm on our rides, sighing deeply with appreciation.

Mariposa lilies dot the prairie grassland. There are also a scattering of tiny pink asters and lavender blue dicks. Most of the oak trees out here have lost their old leaves and are already producing soft grey-green ones. The sun is about to go down so we head back in the direction of the trailers. Helen's dogs, Brindi and Bear, run about the horses' feet, then race down a swell to a cattle tank and splash around. Seen from a distance, I think that Brindi is in some kind of trouble, but the dog simply doesn't know how to swim and tries to paddle in an upright position so that only her head is visible. She manages to make it out of the water and then the dogs run around the tank after harriers.

When the pack returns, Barranca accidentally steps on Bear's foot. Howling, he goes hopping away on three feet. Helen immediately dismounts to comfort her dog, swatting at Brindi to stay away—she doesn't care for this Pit Bull with her crooked tail and heavy breathing. But after some soothing Bear is running beside us again. I'm glad my dogs aren't with us adding to all the commotion.

The sun has now set, and we all make predictions as to where the moon will rise. We believe that it will come up somewhere over the Huachuca Mountains, but we will have to wait and see. It's getting darker and colder by the minute. In March, the sun and moon rise directly across from each other, but now, a month later, as the sun sets further north, the moon will rise further south. None of us can decipher any moon glow.

I am now the only one mounted, and from my high vantage point, I keep thinking that I see a glimmer of light—"Oh look!" No, it's nothing. "There it is!" Nope.

"She's crying moon," Anita laughs.

Only Venus is visible in the dark night sky, crisp and clear, the sinking sun setting off the Patagonia Mountains with a lovely pinkish hue.

Anita and I ride back to the trailers to get her bottle of Pinot Grigio. The horses' hooves spark in the darkness and Saddle Mountain stands out in silhouette. I pick up the long wool coat I have just had cleaned for Helen. It had been so hot this afternoon I didn't think I would need more than a parka vest. Now I am chilled, and the long black coat makes me feel toasty warm and equine elegant.

Back up on the rise, Mason joins us in the Nissan. Anita opens the bottle of wine, passing glasses around. She then cuts some Saga blue cheese to put on crackers. We're all starving. I, for one, have never had wine and cheese on horseback before—*but this is fun!*

There is still no sign of the full moon, not even a glimmer, and I am getting tipsy. It is hard to wait for a moon to appear, sort of like *a watched pot doesn't boil.* Maybe, we have to turn our backs on it. Meanwhile, the horses are happily munching. Green grass is beginning to sprout up everywhere thanks to the glorious winter rains. The horses don't seem to mind the novelty of being out in the dark with half-drunk riders.

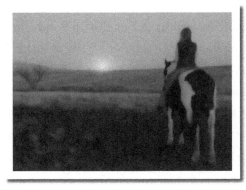

Finally

Finally, Helen is the first one to spot the moon—way down in the direction of Mexico. What a surprise—it is actually nowhere near the Huachucas. Rising over the plain makes the moon's appearance less dramatic than when it rose over the mountains on New Year's Eve. It is now as golden as the sun. "It looks like a peach!" Helen cries, and we are all glad to see it come into view.

We ride back to the horse trailers, Mason transporting our wicker basket filled with food. After loading the horses, we are eager to eat. Anita is especially appreciative that I have brought real linens and a full dinner. We decide on a French picnic out of the back of the car, so that we can see what we are eating—fried chicken, asparagus, potato salad vinaigrette, red wine, and Mint Milanos.

By half past eight, Mason is ready to head home, while the three of us lie down on the ground and look up at the sky, laughing and carrying on as women do when they're together. A multitude of stars have now appeared overhead. Even though the horses rumble around in their trailers, we are relaxed and hoot when a border patrol van goes by—"Hide," I yell. "They'll see us!"

We each have a smoke and puff into the darkness, talking about the art center where Helen teaches. Anita is working on a play with eighteen kids that will be performed in our local Tin Shed. Then, Anita announces that both her father and father-in-law have the same birthdays, and that her mother and mother-in-law both cut off the same index finger while chopping wood. For some reason we find this hilarious.

Helen says that horses sleep in seven-minute segments, and this sounds peculiar but possible, I guess. Where do people get their information? Have our horses dozed off and woken up several times, wondering where they are in the middle of the night while their riders roll around on the ground, delighted by the sight of pristine stars? I have never seen the night sky so clearly.

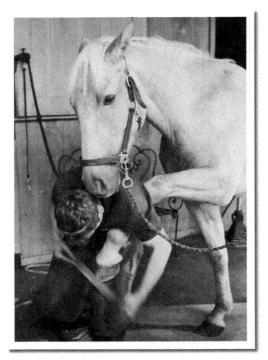

Keith Warner

Keith and Kacy

Keith and Kacy fly into Tucson from Great Barrington, ready to transport my horses back to Massachusetts. Kacy is astounded by how much Peanut has grown over the winter. He is now just as tall as Barranca, perhaps 16.1 hands, but he is still so skinny he doesn't seem like a very imposing horse.

It is a beautiful, sunny day with only a light breeze. All the mesquite trees have leafed out, and wildflowers surround the trails with sweeps of lavender, red, and yellow. The ocotillos have not fully opened their red tips, poised there on the ends of their tall, spindly wands, but soon they will be in full flower.

Down by the Sonoita Creek, the water is low, but there is still some visual refreshment. A large owl takes off in front of us, and later down the trail we see a pair of gray hawks. Coming onto the long narrow trail where the footing is soft and clean, we enjoy several long canters. A great blue heron lifts off downstream.

Keith, my farrier, has not ridden much in the past couple of years. "I'm underneath horses all the time, so I don't have much time to get on top of them," he explains. Back home, Kacy is always trying to get him to ride to no avail, so having him along now is fun for her.

In November, when they made the four-day haul down here with the horses, Keith asked Kacy to marry him out on the front porch of *Casa Durazno*. Now she wears a beautiful engagement ring, and they plan on marrying up at our place on Rose Hill: 09.10.11. That should be easy to remember.

Kacy has been working for me since she was fourteen. Her parents used to drive her up to my barn to muck the stalls, until she got her own car. In her modest, quiet way, she knows more about horses than almost anyone I know. She has won so many blue ribbons that she doesn't even bother to collect them anymore. She is also in charge of the Beinecke barn, *Harmony Hill*, back in South Egremont, Massachusetts, and helps train young riders who want to jump and show, while continuing to take care of my horses when I am away. I feel fortunate to have her and Keith in charge of transporting Barranca and Peanut back East where Rocket is waiting for them. Tonka will stay here in Arizona in a large turnout with many companions, going barefoot until I return.

With his mechanical bent, Keith can fix anything. "He is such a *guy*," I exclaim, as he recounts hunting and fishing tales. Kacy agrees, nodding sweetly. He tells us about some of the games farriers play, including shooting anvils up into the air with explosives.

The sun is intense, and we all agree that we should head back—they have four long days of hauling ahead of them, and I don't want them to be sore or exhausted as they start out. Riding up the arid trail to the parking lot, I notice that in just a few short hours of midday sun, the ocotillos have begun to fully open, as if some higher power with hot chile breath had exhaled on them. The hillsides are now a sweep of red. "We've got to appreciate beauty wherever we can out here," I tell them. This might not be as astonishing as New England's autumnal display, but in Arizona, this is about as good as it gets.

We leave the outside barn lights on that night, as they want to leave for Santa Fe at around 5:00 A.M. when it will still be dark. They should arrive at their first stop no later than 3:00 P.M., and will have the afternoon and evening to explore the city.

I kiss my big boy, Barranca, good night, and begin to have separation anxiety, knowing how much I will miss him during the next three weeks. I whisper to him that soon he will be back in the green fields of the Berkshires, and that he should try to endure the long ride. "Horse Heaven is waiting for you," I tell him. He seems to understand and licks my hand, licks both of them.

It does matter if your horse has a sweet personality. Barranca's loving licks are like kisses. Perhaps he's just searching for salt, but I feel it is heartfelt, especially in contrast to one horse I had years ago.

My dressage trainer at the time convinced me that I should buy this amazing Selle Français-Thoroughbred cross who was 16.3 hands and very well-educated. From the get-go, he pinned his ears back when anyone approached his stall, but my trainer assured me that a lot of horses had that bad habit.

Once I was on him, he seemed nice enough. He had beautiful gaits and could also jump. But when my trainer tried him out, he reared, and she quickly dismounted, as she had already suffered a head injury from a rearing horse and didn't want to get hurt again. Still, I quickly fell for this flea-bitten grey. I named him Nashotah, after a small town in Wisconsin. Having grown up with a difficult mother, I was sure that I could get him to love me if I tried hard enough. But he could never forget whatever it was that had warped his sense of trust.

He developed a foot abscess shortly after I purchased him, and whenever I cross-tied him to dress his wound, he would paw and paw at the rubber mat in the barn. I thought it was an odd habit, but I ignored it, and soon, as he healed, he seemed to paw a bit less, but the ear-pinning continued throughout the rest of his life.

Confused by his behavior, I brought in a horse psychic, and she spent a good deal of time going over him. Without asking me anything about his behavior, she suddenly announced that he had been severely beaten around his legs for pawing in his stall. This had made him defensive. I was amazed. But even given this understanding, there was no changing his behavior. This deep hurt had been stamped into his unforgiving brain, and we never established a heartfelt connection.

It sometimes helps me to remember these things as I try to understand difficult people as well—to know why they act the way they do, and to try and work around it, not to expect too much. All you can do is give. I have found that when someone lashes out at me, it rarely has anything to do with what I have done. I have to remind myself—*don't take it personally*. There is usually something else going on.

Nashotah passed away in his own good time one winter while I was out in Arizona. Kacy took care of him and had him buried at the foot of the pasture. It was only then that I discovered the ease of my cousin Sarah's gaited horses.

I remember riding her well-trained Tennessee Walker one day in the hills of Colrain. We were moving up a steep incline and I could not believe it. "I feel like I'm dreaming," I called back to her. "It's like spreading cream cheese—this is fantastic! He is so smooth!"

Sarah felt that her horses were also more bombproof than most, possibly because they had been used for hunting. I had been dumped too many times by Nashotah. All it took was the appearance of a leaping deer, or a flapping plastic bag, or one of those terrifying "walking birds" (wild turkeys), and then it was as if a car had hit us broadside.

Now, if something alarms Barranca, he stops in his tracks, stock-still, but he doesn't bolt or hurt me. I imagine what it would be like to lose this horse, how bereft I would be, inconsolable. You might think that an animal could never compensate for the lack of human love, but I disagree. A big-hearted animal can be the greatest consolation.

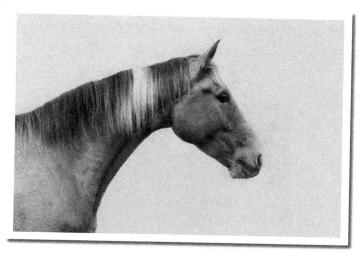

Looking Toward Home

Anxious

Even in my sleep I am anxious about this departure. I wake at four in the morning and go see if the trailer is still in the yard. There it is, lit up by the barn lights. But when I finally get up around seven, it is gone, and I feel a pang—a big hole of absence inside me.

Tonka is probably feeling the same thing, locked into his stall. I know he must be worried, left behind, but he lets me brush him down. Tonka looks off in the direction the trailer took earlier this morning. He whinnies out to his friends, but they are long gone, probably passing into southern New Mexico by now. I lead him over to the pasture across the road, and he goes galloping around the field whinnying and searching for his companions.

When I get back to the house, I give Helen a call, and she offers to let me borrow Bendajo as a companion horse. How wonderful to have an understanding cousin close by. Tonka is thrilled to see a pal arrive, and I am also grateful.

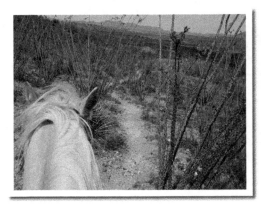

Ocotillo Trail

We Saw Everything!

There is nothing nicer than riding alone on a good horse with a faithful, quiet dog beside you. Bali is a good follower—he instinctively understands the path, and it is a joy to watch him exploring, submerging in the water and then trotting ahead. Here on the Sonoita Creek, I am beginning to feel the heart-tug of departure, soon to leave my beloved Southwest. Tonka is cooperating exceptionally well today, as if he senses he is now my "Number One Horse," and his big-horse-ego likes that—he is responding with great athleticism as well as sweetness.

Tonka also wins the award for the most *poops* per ride. Inevitably he lets loose in the trailer, and I have to kick it out with my boot, but then, out on the trail, he will stop and do his duty seven or eight more times. I figure, better here than in the paddock. I don't know if he is just a "Nervous Nelly," or if he has an exceptionally good digestive system, but right on schedule, he stops and takes another dump.

The ocotillo is now in full flaring bloom, but many of the other wildflowers have passed, with the exception of the "fried egg in the pan" white blooms of the prickly poppy. Their tissue-thin blossoms rest on top of their thistles all along the trail. Nature has its rhythm, as if she didn't want us to go without a visual treat for long—always something orchestrated to entertain the eye.

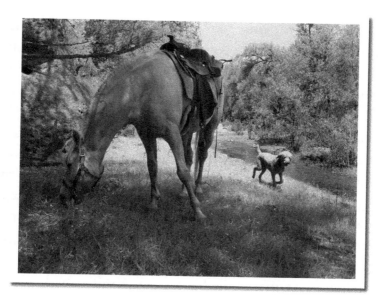

By Sonoita Creek

Tonka is quite familiar with this trail by now, and we move along smoothly until we descend into the creek and our path is blocked by an enormous bull, his massive balls hanging down like gunpowder sacks. But this old fellow is rather sedentary. Perhaps he is a bit of a "Ferdinand" as he munches on fresh green cottonwood leaves, not paying us much attention.

We skirt around him and ride on out to the Indian cave where we normally stop for lunch. It is still early, only 11:30 A.M., but I don't want to tire my dog. So we cross the creek and settle down in the shade, a perfect place to take a break. Tonka is treated to riverside grass, and Bali wanders about in the stream to cool his feet, while I eat my salami-and-cheese sandwich and drink a mango smoothie. The day is dazzling, and the greenery surrounding the creek is a pleasure. I could stay here for hours.

Heading back, I notice how Tonka is always aware of any unusual creature before I am—he makes a miniscule halt and swerves when he sees a coyote standing down below in the running stream. As two separate creatures, we observe each other. And then a hundred yards up the path, I hear a rustling in the leaves and a six-foot-long, red coachwhip snake wriggles up onto the canyon wall. I begin to keep an eye out for rattlers, as the midday heat has increased, and soon they will be a real presence. Little lizards run about on the ground and up the canyon walls. A little further on, Tonka shies when a wild turkey bolts from the underbrush. "Gee," I say out loud, "we're seeing everything today," including some white-tailed deer that bound across the path up ahead.

When we return to the barn, I give Tonka a bath, shampooing his mane and tail. Then I leave him tied to the rail to dry. I offer him a drink from the upright hose and he slurps it up as if it were a bubbler.

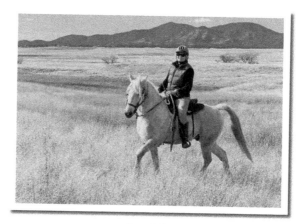

Last Ride

Goodbye San Rafael

Goodbye to the Patagonias. Goodbye to the grey-green, burnt-out grasslands that stretch all the way to Mexico. Goodbye to the transients and the burlap bales dropped along the roadside. Goodbye to the border patrol in their dusty white vans with green stripes. Goodbye to the grand Huachucas. Goodbye to Saddle Mountain, and Indianhead, too, peeking out behind. Goodbye to Red Mountain, that majestic, muscular presence. Goodbye to the border fence with all its problems. Goodbye to the red earthen roads, the desert *agave*, and the stunted oaks that endure the persisting winds. Goodbye to the arid skies, to undisturbed moonlight and brilliant stars. Goodbye to the Herefords huddled by the water tank. Goodbye to barbed wire and those treacherous cattle guards. Goodbye to the lone coyote and the screeching hawk wheeling overhead. Goodbye to this clean sweep of vista that always extends my soul—goodbye Arizona, goodbye—*until we meet again.*

MASSACHUSETTS

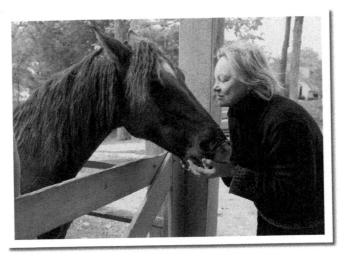

Love Boat

Barn Again

We leave Patagonia, and head up to Scottsdale to say goodbye to my mother. She is now in a rehabilitation facility, but it has become quite clear to my sister, who has just flown in from Wisconsin, that Mom is not going to recover. Our niece, Daphne, is also there and when she tells Gramma they are going to have to move her, Mom says softly, "No hospital, home."

After conferring with the doctors, Cia decides to Med-Vac Mom back to Oconomowoc. The godsend is that she will never have to go into a nursing facility, or live through the terrible end-stage of Alzheimer's.

Years before, in Oconomowoc, Wisconsin, I was with my mother during her first bad hallucination episode. Even though it was way past midnight, my mother was wide awake. She thought that she had been watching a movie—it had been like a waking nightmare.

"There were people all over the room," she said, "hoards of them, Muslims and blacks. And then I was in the cockpit of some Army plane, flying over a place like Siberia. It was so wintry and cold, and there were battleships and rooms and rooms of brothels, with men doing things to each other, beating up women, hurting small children. It was terrible, so icy and cold, and then there was this palatial hotel where they had everything you could ever want, crocodile bags that would normally cost $3,000 were only about $700, and linens you would not believe—everything, so many luxuries!" It sounded like a vision of hell.

"There's a man standing behind you!" she pointed. "He's ugly with wild red hair and pock marks all over his face. Tell him to get out of here!" She was so convincing, I swung around to look. "And there are children peeling the wallpaper! Why are they doing that? Daphne is destroying the lampshade. Tell her to stop it! Why are there so many people in my room? They are being very rude, sticking their tongues out."

"Your mind is just playing tricks on you, Mom."

"Don't lie to me! I know what I'm seeing. And there's water streaming down the walls, look." She held out her hand as if she could feel it. "And what is this tissue—it's falling from the ceiling." I looked in her hand as if I could see it too, but of course there was nothing there.

Mom insisted that there were women in the closet stealing Popi's clothing.

"No, there aren't any women," I said.

"I know what I see!"

"Okay, let's get up and go over there." I helped her get out of bed and led her over. She looked perplexed, rattling through my father's naked wooden hangers. She agreed that the women had left. At least they weren't sitting in Bluebeard's closet with pools of clotted blood.

"Let me rub your feet," I suggested, trying to soothe her with the rose-scented oil I'd brought from home. I sang her the songs that she used to sing to me in my childhood, "Summertime" and "Mighty Like a Rose." In a pathetic little voice, she tried to sing along with me, sometimes leaning up on her elbow to see what else was going on.

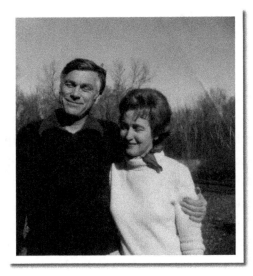

Mom and Dad

The next morning, downstairs, Mom's hallucinations continued—"There are those same children, standing in the hallway, with a big tall black man. What do you think they want?" She motioned them in, waving with her hand, with an endearing, welcoming expression on her face.

Mom insisted that this was not her home, and she wanted to get in the car with Wanda and go back home immediately. "I don't like this hotel," she said.

"This isn't a hotel," I assured her. "You're staying in your own house, Broadoaks." I encouraged her to come outside and sit down on the lawn chair beneath the pergola, before her round English garden.

Often, in the past, she and Wanda could be seen here weeding, or planting, side-by-side, both of them in broad, straw hats.

"Let me read you a story," I said to her and she nodded her head, content for a moment. It was nice reading out loud to my mother. I liked this reversal, taking care of her, but soon the hallucinations took hold again. "Why are those children destroying my plants?"

"They aren't destroying anything. You're seeing things."

"They're using clippers. They're tearing at the flowers with scissors. Why are they doing that?"

"Just close your eyes and listen."

As I read, she began to calm down. She told me that my story was, "Very well written. You are an excellent writer." She had always said that. She had always been supportive of me in that realm, even when I was ten years old and read her each new chapter from "Betsy and Pixie Ride Again," my first handwritten book, composed on a notepad of yellow paper.

She wanted iced tea, and Wanda brought her a full tumbler. "Wanda knows how to do everything." Mom was more dependent on Wanda than on any of us.

At odd moments, Mom seemed lucid, and continued to surprise me—coming around a corner like a burst of sunlight emerging from a cloud, only to open her arms and beam—"You know I love you, Laura."

Lost on a sea of forgetfulness, she could still touch bottom sometimes. I felt more like a shipwrecked person. How easily people say it—I love you, I love you...just tossed off. How rarely it's said with true feeling.

I thought of my mother, my father's wife, who wrote love letters to him overseas, day after day, full of passion, always unwavering. She only thought the best of him now. "He was such a wonderful husband," even if she couldn't remember his name. "He was always so much fun."

"You had your difficult times," I reminded her.

"Really, I don't remember that, when?"

"Oh, when he'd go off riding with other people."

"Oh yes," she laughed, "he did do that." She no longer seemed to care.

When my father was asked, "What was the most fortunate thing that ever happened to you?" he answered, "Marrying my wife."

Conflicted, unsure, often secretive, I was my father's daughter—grandiose, yet somehow dwarfed. Was I standing in for him now? I would send my mother lilies and chocolate. I could forgive her jealous heart. Still, at least, I could say it, right? "I love you too, Mom," and mean it. I could come around, and embrace her, finally receiving her love.

On saying goodbye to my mother for what would be the last time, I consider forgiving her for not being a very good mother, but instead, I apologize for not always being a good daughter. She accepts that. We have reconciled over the years since my father's death, but I still can't conjure up the emotions you're supposed to feel when your mother is dying. I feel rather empty.

It is a short five-hour flight to Newark, and soon we are picked up by our trusty driver and are off to the Berkshires.

As we go, I feel disoriented. The landscape hurts my eyes—*too green*. Everything looks too close, not enough space. It is hot and humid. But when we pull in our driveway, I am happy to see Barranca, Peanut, and Rocket out in their enormous field. Do they know how lucky they are? And how little they would have to graze upon if they were still in Arizona?

I don't ride on the first day back but wait until the following morning to saddle up Barranca. I take him out on the familiar trails behind the house. We have miles and miles of trails here—most of them on our neighbor's lumber land—but many trees have fallen across the paths during the course of the winter, and I am annoyed by all the blockages. We work our way around the debris and head down to Long Pond. But I still don't feel like I'm "home." The lilacs are out in abundance, dripping with moisture, and Barranca moves out beautifully, but I am in an off-mood, not even entranced by the wild lavender phlox that is springing up along the trails.

The next morning, I take Peanut out for a go, and he surprises me with his willing, fast walk. I treat his mouth with utmost gentleness. The trick will be teaching others how to handle him so that he doesn't get confused or sour from varied communications.

Meanwhile, my sister and I exchange emails and phone calls about our mother, back in Wisconsin. One day, she seems to be doing fine, and the next, she barely opens her eyes. She is in a comfortable hospital bed, facing the lake, and seems content for the most part. She still seems to recognize people, and beams at Mary Read, my cousin's wife, one of her favorites, though when my brother David arrives, she asks, "Are you mine?"

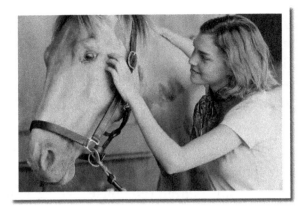

Arizona Muse

Baldwin Hill

Baldwin Hill Farm, just fifteen minutes away, is another world of wide open fields on top of a gentle rise. This is where we first lived when we came to the Berkshires, when Ayler was only two years old. We rented the Burdsall farmhouse with its four-hundred acres, and I rode all over this hill with Bunny Kirchner, an eighty-year-old, mad-for-horses local man. I know the trails here well.

During Bunny's last few years, he lived in an ambulance. Whenever we dropped by his emergency vehicle, it was disturbing to see the deep trash on the floor. Sometimes, when I sent Ayler in to deliver food, he was afraid that Bunny was dead. But Bunny lived into his nineties, and kept on riding right up to the end. Horses were his passion.

Bunny was an old-timer who knew everything about every family who lived along the road. But he often did things in a strange manner, like using a knife to cut a slit in my girth, rather than using a hole-punch. One day when I was riding his stallion and we took off at a gallop, the burst of energy straining against the leather made the girth snap, and I went flying, banging my head on the hard gravel road. Now I always wear a helmet.

My young friend, Arizona Muse, and I proceed to the crossroads on Baldwin Hill and follow the tractor trails that go from one field to the next to the next. There is a sweet expansiveness up here that one does not feel in the closed-in forest—*it lifts my spirits.*

Now that Arizona's baby Nikko is getting older, she is considering getting back into modeling. At twenty-one, she thinks she is too old, but her agency, NEXT, is thrilled to have her return. She has her willowy figure back and a lot of jobs seem to be coming her way. I tell her to watch out and not scratch her face. Arizona is so beautiful, it is almost difficult to take her in—a natural perfection that is dazzling, and yet she seems grounded, confident, and very assured for someone so young.

We ride up to the little Egremont Cemetery and down the dump road until we find an opening into another set of fields. Now, we ride quietly and just take all of this in. So often, it is better not to talk on horseback but to try and remain in touch with what is happening with your horse, how the bit feels in his mouth, how he is walking on the path—giving leg signals and making subtle moves.

Arizona and I both appreciate the great silence that surrounds us.

She is getting the hang of the four-beat gait, and is a lot more relaxed about her son, who is now with her mother, Davina. Last year, while Arizona was still nursing, she paid more attention to the clock when we rode. The tug of the mother-nursing-baby bond was always there, putting her on remote alert, but now neither of us wears a watch, for we are in a timeless zone of pure pleasure.

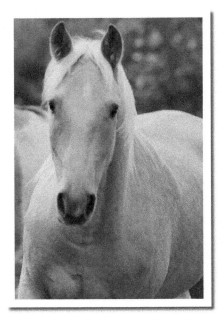

Rocket Man

Familiar Territory

I ride Barranca alone through the woods and then up the Sarsaparilla Highway. This woodland trail is surrounded by thin, dark-skinned, birch-like trees, and if you break off a twig and give it a chew, it tastes vaguely like root beer. Climbing the narrow switchback trail, we head to the top of the mountain, zigzagging back and forth—good for the horses' haunches.

While I ride, I think about my mother at my sister's house in Wisconsin and wonder if I should go out there. Cia assures me that I don't need to come. The hospice workers have said that Mom only has another day or two to live. That is hard to believe. I keep wondering when I will feel something.

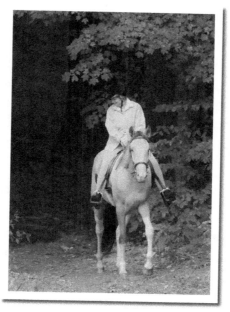

Elizabeth Beautyman

Riding in the Rain

Last night, I woke three times gasping for air, a kind of sleep apnea I rarely experience. The second time, I felt a dark brown presence by my bed, which I struck out at with my hand. Turning on the light, getting my wind back, I wondered if it related to my mother's struggle for oxygen, as she had begun "Cheyne-Stokes" breathing. Was this a visitation of some sort?

It is raining this morning when I awake so I figure that my ride with Elizabeth will be cancelled. But she calls and says that she is still game to go out, so we decide to take our chances. The rain does let up, but the wind through the leaves sends showers down upon us. When I break a branch overhead and she gets sprayed, she yells out, "*Hey!*" Don't do that.

"Sorry," I answer. It is a compulsive habit I have, always clearing the trails overhead, snapping branches. Helen's ex-husband, the psychologist, liked to say that breaking branches indicated anger. Helen and I always laughed over that, snapping away.

I take Elizabeth down to Long Pond. The trail is slippery going downhill—we leave horse-hoof skid marks all along the way. Once we are on solid ground, we enjoy a few good canters, and she gets the feel for Peanut's moves. It is a stormy morning with thundershowers coming and going, but that only adds to our excitement—*all those negative ions.*

That evening, I hear one of the horses ringing the tall standing bell by the corral. I assume it is Peanut, my trickster. Horses have an innate sense of timing and love a regular schedule. I guess it is time to walk them down to their field for the evening. Rising from the comfortable love seat, I hear the phone ring. It is my sister. Quietly she says, "Mom just went. You were my first call."

I sit on the love seat in silence, thinking of what Phil Caputo said after his father died last winter, how it was like looking up at a familiar landscape and the mountain that had always been there, was suddenly gone.

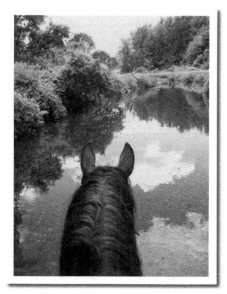

Alford Brook

Summer Fields

With the sun shining through the clouds, the air is at that perfect temperature. I ride Barranca out into the fields, which exude such a sweet smell of earth and grass, I feel intoxicated. We wade through the Alford Brook, climbing up a bank, proceeding uphill into more open pasture.

A few years ago, my horse Nashotah balked when I urged him into this field, but I made him move forward. And then, I saw a big black dog at a distance and yelled out, "*Go on, big dog, go home.*" But the "big dog" stood up on its hind legs. It was a BEAR! No wonder Nashotah had almost refused to enter this field, for bears have a very pungent smell, like rotting meat, quite unpleasant to horses. Luckily, we got out of there before Nashotah took the bit in his mouth and bolted.

But now, we pass through the field undisturbed and head into the deep woods. The deerflies aren't too bad. In fact, Barranca shakes off his bright blue, net ear-covering, and I tuck it into my pocket. There is the faint smell of grape on the road home, followed by fresh tar, and then mown fields. It is so mild and blissful, Barranca so easy in hand, that I feel I could almost fall asleep in the saddle. *Somnambulistic.*

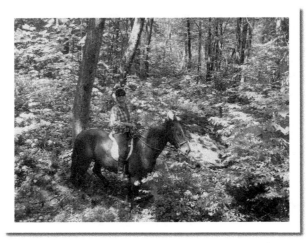

Mountain Laurel

Mount Washington

Betsy Spears and Christopher Bamford live at the end of Mount Washington Road. It is a long haul uphill, but a welcomed change from the normal known. Today, Betsy wants to take me up her dirt road to see the voluminous mountain laurel that blooms wild along the roadside in pale pink and subtle rose. The bushes spread back into the forest like a fairyland.

Heading back into the woods, I note how it has a sylvan medieval feel to it. A small stream runs alongside the path with large rock outcroppings covered in moss. The forest here is like nature's chapel, flickering with bird song and filtered light. Riding beside the stream, I imagine these ravines filled with turbulent water when the winter snows melt, but now it is simply flowing along at a soothing pace.

The trails are all well-marked, but few riders have come this way, apparently, as many branches hang rather low. She ducks under while I try to prune a bit as we go, *snap, snap*.

On the path, we meet a solitary hiker who says that the stone boulders on top of the mountain have rattlesnakes right now. It is breeding season, and they are coming out. Betsy and Chris found two large rattlesnakes behind their barn this morning. A local snake man caught them in a garbage can, marking their rattles so that their movement could be tracked for a local study—funny to come from the land of desert reptiles and to feel their presence right here in the Berkshires.

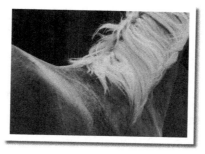

Double Mane

Kacy, Regular Rocket Rider

Luckily, Rocket has not been stumbling this year. Perhaps, he has outgrown that awkward adolescent phase where his limbs were not quite connected to his brain.

This morning, Kacy and I trailer over to Mountain Road. If my memory serves me right, there is a long path up here that runs along the crest of the ridge through abundant woods. We find it easily enough. Soon, we are in forest wilderness with birds singing all about us. It is a lovely day to be riding, getting a scent of juniper and sweet fern that smells mildly like peppermint when crushed by the horses' hooves.

Maneuvering around a steel cable meant to keep out cars, we pass a handmade sign that says CARDIAC HILL. Several doctors own this tract of land, and they have done some clearing since the days when I used to ride here with Ayler on his New Forest pony. Ayler always liked exploring new areas, and we often snuck onto private land. Once, we were chased by a farmer in his beat-up truck. We knew all the hiding spots, the getaway paths, and we were never caught. One land owner, fed up with us, posted a sign, "*NO WHORS RIDING.*"

The biggest difference between riding in the East and the West is that Arizona has so much public land that you have easy access to almost every possible trail. Even ranchers, who lease land from the government, don't mind you riding through as long as you close all gates behind you. But here we are often trespassing, sneaking around. One neighbor created big branch barricades to keep me out and even went so far as to hide broken bottles along the trail I used. I don't ask permission because I'm afraid of being told, "No." My father's friendly method of persuasion was—*if I am stopped, I will talk my way out of it.*

I don't believe the cardiac doctors are anywhere around. They mostly come here for hunting season, so we have these wild woods to ourselves today. Passing several marsh ponds coated with algae, we hear the deep croak of bullfrogs. What a great place for birders. But then as I'm day-dreaming,

Barranca almost steps into a rotted-out metal culvert hole. That could have been a disaster. Horrified, I yell back to Kacy, "Watch out!"

I remember the terrible accident Donna's horse Zwen had when he stepped through a rusty culvert like this and sawed up his leg. At the time, everyone in the barn thought he should be put down, but Doctor Hammond and the stable groom, Pinky, saved his life. The great Dutch Warmblood survived the trauma and is still Donna's beloved pet.

One tragedy reminds me of another, and I think of Cody trapped in that cattle guard. It's hard to imagine his panic and pain.

I tell Kacy about giving up Ayler's little pony, Star, one autumn day when my son had outgrown her, and how Cody whinnied desperately after her, staring in her departing direction. After hours of calling out, he hung his head and became depressed for the rest of the winter. How thoughtless of me to deprive him of his beloved companion. I'm convinced that horses do fall in love, and they too can suffer heartbreak.

On our way back to the trailer, I dismount, and go to gather branches to plug up the treacherous hole. This should mark it for future rides. When we reach the chain that marks off this private land, I smile at the hand-scribbled sign: "No Trespassing. Surveillance cameras in operation. You will be prosecuted!" Good luck.

WISCONSIN

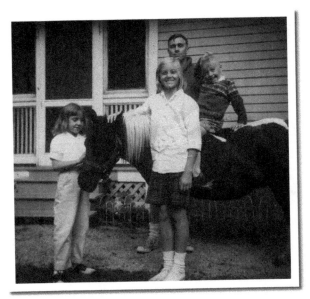

By the Cottage

Lake Country

Returning to Oconomowoc for our mother's funeral, I greet family from all over the country. Even Clovis and his wife and their two small sons, Kailer and Cash, have come all the way from Australia.

Every time Kailer sees me, he cries out, *"HI GRAMMA!"* It is enough to melt my heart. I realize, since my mother passed away, I am the only "Gramma" in our immediate family now, and I love the title—it doesn't make me feel old.

The little boys love to walk over to the farm to look at the horses and feed the chickens. They never seem to tire of gathering those delightful, warm eggs, placing them in the grey cardboard carton, counting them up. I should also count my blessings.

But coming back here to the scene of my childhood, a lot of memories surface and they aren't all nice.

When we gathered for my father's last birthday party, he was in the middle of radiation treatment and Mom was at her worst. She didn't like the focus being all on him, and she didn't like so many people in her house. When I arrived, I asked if I could stay in the "pink room."

"But that's a nice room, why don't you stay in the..."

Why shouldn't I stay in a nice room?

Then one morning, while helping myself to some orange juice out of the fridge, she came raging into the kitchen and grabbed the carton out of my hands, spraying it everywhere, screaming, "That's not for you—it's for your father!"

I grabbed it back and yelled at her, "Why are you always so mean to me?"

She hit me, and I struck her back. My niece, little Isabelle, was cringing, and my son, Clovis, dragged me away. But I'd had it with her! HAD IT.

Once when I was visiting Oconomowoc, we were all sitting around a large, round table at the Lake Club, and I asked Mom if I could have a bite of her Schaum torte, my favorite, not wanting to order a full portion for myself. She turned on me and announced over the table, "You should be losing five pounds a week." Good idea, in a matter of months I wouldn't exist.

I think about when my parents were passing through New York and I wanted to have a meal with them—my mother's response was, "This is our time to be alone together, Laura. We're only seeing the people we really want to see."

But finally, I have grown tired of my own processing, tired of opening old wounds. Isn't it time to heal them, let them go? I have so many good memories of those summer months—building forts in the horse field with leftover fence poles, organizing rodeos, running our putt-putts through the canals where we hid out on secret islands. We had picnic lunches down on the dock, and watched the sunfish slithering beneath the white planks of the pier as we fed them bits of Wonderbread.

I really liked our family dinners over at the big house where there was a painted mural of pheasants running all around the room. The cousins would try to out-eat each other, piling up ears of baby bantam corn, sprinkling sugar on thick-sliced tomatoes from our voluminous garden. There were popovers with homemade currant jelly—each jar with a little wax lid—and Winnie, our grandmother's cook, always had frosted ginger cookies for us if we were willing to listen to her. Even our rather aloof grandfather allowed us to drop saccharin pills into his coffee as we chanted, "Swimming swimming swimming swimming," while they dissolved.

But best of all was riding with Gramma. "Uphill fast, downhill slow, on the level let them go." She was a fearless rider and took off when we hit the edge of a shorn field. I only worried if we'd be able to stop the stampede when we came to the end—a boundary of tall, dense corn.

My mother could not abide my grandmother, and she mistrusted my boyfriend, Kenny Buchanan, the "bad boy" of the lake. I think she was afraid that he would knock me up, but we never went beyond first base.

Of course now I want to ride over to Kenny's old summer house where we first learned how to kiss. I know it is time to let my negative memories go, and what better way to do that than to go for a ride? Eager to get out alone by myself, I decide to try out Daphne's new horse, Booker, a Friesian/Quarter Horse cross.

"He needs a strong rider," Daphne warns me, for he is an eight-year-old powerhouse.

Still, I am eager to try him. Over at the stable, the farmhand is wiping Booker down with bug spray. The deerflies here can be terrible. Seeing this majestic bay horse standing cross-tied, I realize how huge he is. I know he bucked off my cousin, Ross, this spring, so I feel a bit apprehensive, but go ahead and throw on his Western saddle. He stands nicely while I mount, but I can feel his nervous energy as we leave the other horses and head down the road.

Passing the tennis court, I ask the players if they could hold the ball for a moment while I pass, for Booker seems spooky. The driveway is now paved, rather than dirt as it was in our childhood. I keep giving him leg signals to move him forward, stroking his neck and praising him constantly. I know he has not been ridden much, and he is clearly herd-bound, but he does seem willing to please.

We continue down Pettit Road to the old Buchanan driveway. The woods here are dense, and the deerflies nest in Booker's mane, annoying him. They even bite my thighs, but I want to find that lovely riding trail that goes down to the lakefront and around the point.

In the fall, the oak leaves here are a dazzling yellow against the autumnal blue. I find the hidden path and ride down to the lapping shore, still reluctant to canter, but I do get into a nice spongy jog. I don't want Booker taking off with me so I keep him in check, but it is tiring holding him back.

Heading home, as soon as we leave the Buchanan's driveway and turn onto Pettit Road, a car goes racing by—*too* fast—unnerving! I'm glad it didn't come up behind me just moments before and feel relieved to get back to the stable without a major incident.

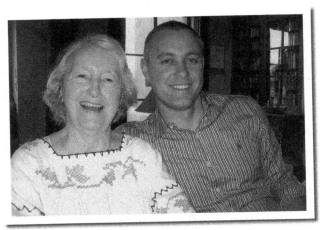

Gramma and Clovis

The next day the funeral is held in a beautiful wooden chapel at the Nashotah Mission. Cia speaks about Mom's Catholic/Jewish heritage, Ayler plays "Hallelujah" on guitar, and then Clovis, Gramma's oldest grandchild, reads some amusing anecdotes from his laptop. But what I remember best is what Abigail wrote about Gramma's last few days.

When we brought Gramma back home, she lay facing the lake, her room filled with flowers. We would take turns sitting with her even when she slept, so that she was never alone. She recognized faces still, and would light up any time we would come in..."Oh, Abigail!" I remember her saying.

One day, my giant Great Dane mix snuck into the room after me and stuck his big, wet nose in her face. I thought she might be alarmed and would shoo him away, but instead she laughed and gave his big, dark head a hug. "Oh my, but who are YOU?!"

We spent those last days singing to her and reading to her and crying with her as she began to understand she was dying. It was an amazing thing to be able to grieve with her, tell her stories, paint her fingernails, and just sit by her side. I'm glad she was able to be at home. It felt like an appropriately dignified departure for Gramma. She got to go, watching the familiar light on Oconomowoc Lake, surrounded by people that loved her.

MASSACHUSETTS

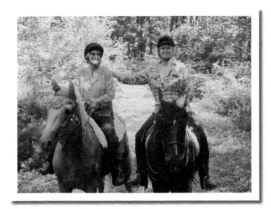

Betsy and Laura

Heat Wave

Betsy and I amble up the ridge looking for a breeze. The morning warmth is comfortable, like loose swaddling on the skin, but we know in a couple of hours it will almost be inhumane to remain on horseback. Heat and flies coupled with high humidity is hard on the horses. Even now, they climb, and stop, and huff and puff.

I wonder what it must be like to be completely covered in fur. How does the cool water feel on their legs and backs after a ride? I spray them down and scrape them off as Betsy mucks. Barranca whips me once with his tail and it stings my face. Does he think I'm another bug?

The horses stay in their stalls all day to escape the heat and flies. Their urine makes the sawdust rank. That evening I run the horses down to the lower field in my golf cart—the lazy way of moving my herd. With Barranca and Peanut on lead ropes, trotting along beside me in the dusk light, the air is fragrant with honey-sweet hedgerows. Rocket barrels down the slope with his white mane flying and they fall into the pasture together, but there are still swarms of flies awaiting them. They run to take cover in the shed with its hanging burlap that shields them from these pests. Why is it so easy to fool a fly?

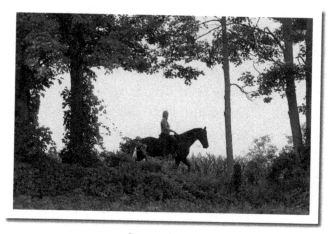

Between Trees

Love at First Sight

I think about the abuse so many people inflict on poor, innocent animals, and how much affection I get from my horses and dogs. In choosing my animals, I have relied on instinct rather than rational pros and cons.

I remember when I first saw Barranca in Scottsdale and how it was love at first sight. Sometimes, while riding, I swear he knows what I'm thinking without my giving him any commands. One day, going down the Alford Road toward our driveway, where we always turned to go back up to the barn, I had another thought—I wanted to ride past and go up a forest trail. I would have expected him to take the turn at the drive, but without my doing anything, he just continued going in the direction I had in mind. This would not have been so remarkable, except for *every other time we had* always turned in at the driveway.

I fell in love with Peanut over the Internet. When I lost Nashotah, my Selle Français, I imagined a young Tennessee Walker gelding, a caramel-and-cream-colored pinto. I didn't even know if such a thing existed, but then there he was at a small breeding barn in Texas. He remained with his mother until he was weaned. Then, at six months old, he was shipped back to Massachusetts. People along the way fell in love with his amber eyes. He was a household pet for a couple of years before he was fully ground-trained. Then he became a docile and excellent ride.

I also had a similar attraction to Tonka Waken at Big Sky Fox Trotters in Scottsdale. Was it just his long Indian-pony forelock and his stud-proud neck, his pale palomino coloring and perfect conformation? I only rode Tonka for half-an-hour before I decided that he had to come back to Patagonia with me. Am I a polygamist when it comes to horses? I'd be happy with Barranca as my only horse, but a solitary equine is rarely happy.

While riding, memories so often surface and percolate. I wonder where these odd thoughts come from, similar to the musings of a twilight reverie, arriving like unexpected house-guests. Images arise oblivious to order, and family members appear as if to remind us that they will inhabit us forever.

I remember Popi yelling down the hallway—"Who stole my scissors?" His large, warm hands and wide, flat fingernails.

I remember Mom knitting me a dark blue sweater. There were many mistakes, but I was quite pleased with it.

I remember him insisting on everyone ordering soup when he took us out to dinner.

I remember her beautiful skin, the thick white cream she put on her face before bed every evening. I wondered if it got on her pillow.

I remember Popi slapping my thigh when we would take off in the car. He'd raise his voice and say, "We're OFF."

I remember the look of glee when Popi and Clovis released a bunch of piglets from the back of his Buick into the middle of a party down by the lake.

I remember her thinking that the subject of horses was "totally boring."

I remember him teasing, "Who's your favorite uncle?!" as he threatened to push a cousin into the lake.

I remember Mom painting our names in the changing room, using her coral-pink fingernail polish.

I remember coming into Broadoaks one morning, asking, "Where is Popi?" He was standing outside with three of his granddaughters, Abigail, Isabelle, and Daphne. There was a little black bat on the side of a tree, and they were trying to feed it bacon.

I remember her helping me organize "sprinkler parties" for the neighborhood kids. Coming from the South, she let us drink Coke.

I remember her saying, "Modulate," when she wanted us to lower our voices.

I remember his cutting our toenails, having us line up for "Dr. Chester."

I remember her loving to rhyme—"We don't smoke and we don't chew and we don't go with the boys who do."

I remember him stopping at the "camel tree" on Buchanan Drive. The tree had a curved trunk and saddle bump, and he would let us play there for as long as we liked.

I remember him feeding the Lipizzans sugar when the sign said clearly not to.

I remember her sitting on the martini boat reading religious tomes, claiming she was now a Born Again Christian. That didn't last.

I remember her napping with all the shades drawn, and how it revived her.

I remember him letting me steer the car when I was too small to reach the pedals.

I remember how she cried when she dropped me off at college. I was surprised by her emotion.

I remember him running in the dark, down the long white pier, diving into Oconomowoc Lake with a tremendous splash.

I remember her telling us to be home when the streetlights came on.

I remember him waking me early to see the herons at Horicon Marsh. The best part of the trip was when the leader, Mrs. Oehlenschlaeger, gave me a miniature wooden chest-of-drawers.

I remember her organizing a birthday party for herself and all of the guests were men.

I remember her favoring my baby brother, David. He got to ride in a flimsy car seat with a plastic steering wheel.

I remember Popi pretending to be out of gas, pumping the pedal, when he was taking a friend of mine home from the movies, telling Mary Allis, "You'll have to walk the rest of the way." I knew he was teasing, but she did not.

I remember her cupboard of long, narrow shoes, how she hid her breasts if I surprised her in the bathtub.

I remember him honking in the tunnel before the Pig n' Whistle, because it made a nice echoing sound, and we encouraged him to do it—Honk, HONK!

I remember her sitting on the green vinyl chaise on the screened-in porch, paging through endless magazines, waiting for my father to come home.

I remember her taking us to the Okauchee Station where Popi would arrive by train, and we'd put pennies on the tracks to flatten them.

I remember him stopping at Kit's Custard when we drove out to the country on Highway 16. I always got a vanilla cone—my older brother told me that was not a real flavor.

I remember the Magic Marker drawings on his emaciated chest, left there after radiation treatment.

I remember her choking, repeatedly, getting the Heimlich maneuver, asserting, "I have a very small opening, Laura."

I remember him walking down the Grand Canyon when Clovis and Ayler and I rode mules. He weighed too much to ride. When he finally made it to Phantom Ranch at the bottom, he was wobbly from dehydration.

I remember Mom taking me into the cabin bathroom at Pike's Peak to show me a twelve-inch-long brown log in the toilet bowl. I was impressed.

I remember him wiping the horses down with bug repellent, sponging them with warm water after a ride. He took such pleasure in it.

I remember the picture of a naked girl on a horse he had hanging in the tack room. To see the nude, you had to flip the decent, dressed version around. Mom got rid of that, along with others of glamorous men nestling their wind-tossed Arabians.

I remember his watch going off in church and him letting it buzz for a very long time. If he sang, he sang extra loud just to attract attention. He would rather have been out riding.

I remember him saying that Mom had the most beautiful shoulders and that I had the Chester legs. Well, thanks.

I remember her taking me shopping for clothes, picking out a brown print dress, which I loved.

I remember him coming up the Carriage House steps, the bang of the baby gate, walking down the hall, clapping his hands together when he had a scoop to deliver, his hope for a good, strong cup of coffee.

I remember the first llama he gave to my brother as a wedding present. It was incredibly soft, and we fed him from a bottle. The llama imprinted on humans and started knocking people down as llamas mate in the prone position.

I remember her obsession for tennis and how she repeatedly told me, "You'd be so good if you only played," even though we were already playing.

I remember him hitting a ball so hard when I was standing at the net that it struck me in the forehead, and I was shy on the court ever after.

I remember him riding in laced-up hiking boots with his feet dangerously deep in the stirrups, the cuffs to his blue jeans turned up high.

I remember her knowledge of English antiques, and how proud she was of her store, though most of Milwaukee preferred reproductions.

I remember him purchasing junk just to be buying something. "Supporting the economy," was his excuse.

I remember her large, pop-bead pearls, and her pink-and-green mumu. She looked very comfortable in it.

I remember him in his red-and-blue striped sweater. He wore it for over a decade. After he died, I put it in the washer, thinking it was cotton, and it shrank.

I remember her grinding up a huge array of pills with a mortar and pestle and eating the powder from a plastic container of apple sauce.

I remember seeing the video of her singing "Happy Birthday" to herself a few days before her passing.

I remember him saying, "Good morning pigeons."

I remember him almost blissful in death, very peaceful, a very graceful parting. It looked so easy. He made everything look easy.

I wonder what they would remember and what I have chosen to forget.

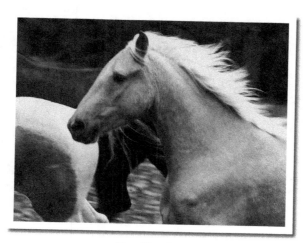

Close Together

Burst of Energy

I'm in a cleaning mood today and tackle the tack room, taking out the old coil rug and pug doormat, shaking them out, sweeping into all the corners, rearranging the baskets and buckets of horse medication, tossing out junk—all super-fluous items—filling the water buckets after giving them a good scrub, doing some deep mucking (careful to bend my knees), tossing a layer of nice fresh shavings into the stalls, putting out fresh hay and sweeping up. It feels good to have everything so neat and tidy. But why can't it stay that way?

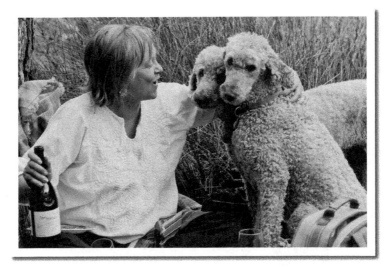

Bali and Cello

New Trail

It is a morning to hold your breath—*that perfect*—clear blue skies and radiant sun through cool, bug-free air. It is so good, so blissfully vibrant it is almost heart-breaking, like new love, when it hurts because it's so terribly fleeting.

Always thrilled to find a new place to ride, this morning Elizabeth and I follow an offshoot from the Mountain Road

Trail. Taking a right uphill, we ride for miles through pure Berkshire forest. Oddly, apples are already falling from the trees, and the horses know it. Goldenrod is up, everything coming early this year. I hope that means an early winter and that I will get to ride in the snow before returning to Patagonia.

We follow the trail as it begins to descend, eating blackberries as we go, plucking the dark ripe fruit from thorny vines. Suddenly, there is an opening, and we have a glorious lookout over the Alford Valley. I assume that we will end up on West Road, but as we continue, almost down to the valley floor, the trail bends to the right and begins to mount again.

We hear the *hoot* of an owl deep in the woods, and it sounds so lonely, haunting.

Both dogs are with us today, and it is turning into a very long ride. I wonder if this is too much for ten-year-old dogs. Marcello is slightly pigeon-toed so it can be more difficult for him to keep up. Bali is my athlete.

"You're lucky your dogs don't go racing after squirrels," Elizabeth says. "They're being awfully good."

"Do you hear that, boys? You're being *awfully good!*"

But then, as we head up a smaller path that will loop us back to the beginning, I realize that Marcello isn't following us. He is nowhere to be seen. Maybe, he took a shortcut back to the trailer. We turn and try to find him, but then in the thick of the forest I hear a pack of coyotes howling over a kill. I am horrified. Have they attacked Marcello? I call out for him, over and over, but no response.

We head back to the gravel road that will take us down to the trailer, and there is Marcello standing with a group of people and two stopped cars. They chew me out for letting my dog run loose out on the road, but I am so happy to see him, I only say, "*Where in the world did you go?*"

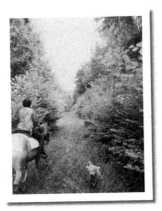

Riding with Betsy Spears

Riding the Same Loop Backward

Barranca is showing signs of the slobbers, and Betsy is appalled. "I've never seen anything like this," she says, as he drools some more. "Do you think it's safe to ride him?"

The slobbers can dehydrate a horse—that is the main risk. It is often a reaction to a fungus that is found on clover. I am suspicious of the new hay we just received, but it could also be something in our own fields. *Slobber!*

I think he will be fine, as long as he has plenty of fresh water to drink along the way, and the trail we'll take has a rushing stream coming off the mountain.

Betsy has to get to a doctor's appointment by one o'clock so she follows me over to the trailhead in her own car while I drive the truck. We are going to take this new path in reverse to see which direction we prefer. As we get on our way, Betsy points out sprays of tiny purple-black elderberries, and we talk about making jam.

As we continue climbing up the trail, Barranca throws a shoe. I hear the telltale clink of metal and hop off to collect it, *yup*, his right front shoe. I check my cell phone to see if there is any reception up here, and I am able to contact Kacy, who calls Keith, my farrier. He can come over later this afternoon. *What service.*

Back at the trailer, I take everything out of my saddle pack—unlock the truck and load the horses. Betsy takes off in her car, and suddenly I cannot find my keys. I do not see them anywhere. Will I have to ride Barranca home leading Peanut all the way? And what about the dogs on the road? People drive so fast and don't slow down for animals. I begin to panic, climbing back in with the horses to check the saddle pack—empty. I dump out the contents of my purse—nothing. Then check all around both seats, front and back and under, until... something *clicks*—my keys are there in the door to the truck.

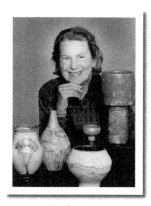

Emily Rose

Fallen Timber

I take my mother-in-law Em a glass of lavender lemonade. She is sitting in her library asleep, but she awakes at my arrival and takes a sip of the drink. Immediately she makes a sour face—*not for her.* So I drink the rest of it down, *yum,* and remind her that her birthday is right around the corner—only ten days away. On the fifteenth of August she will be one-hundred-and-one years old, and we will have a big family potluck in her honor.

I have already ordered her white orchids with little butterfly--shaped blooms, but this afternoon I pick her a bunch of pinks and yellows and blues from the garden. When I present the bouquet, she says softly, "*I will enjoy this forever.*"

Nancy Beach, one of her caregivers, stands by me. We both try to decipher what Em says, but her sense of language has retreated to another world where she seems to slip back and forth over some invisible edge. "*Is she going,*" Em whispers in a very hushed voice. "*Is she going?*"

I lift her from behind into a standing position, and she is able to maneuver her walker back to bed. Then, I head off to ride Barranca. I know a big storm is coming. You can feel it in the air, the humidity and the clouds building up to a sodden, oppressive density.

But Barranca and I have enough time to try out the back trails all the way down to the bottom of Rose Hill. There is a massive set of logs blocking the path. As I look down toward the brook, there are other gigantic trees felled from age and wind, the base of their root systems tipped, exposing the earth that once held them in place. A few of these magnificent trees are probably over a hundred years old, and the loss of them in the forest reminds me of the passing of great personalities who are also felled by time. Emily Rose will be like one of these honorable trees, one of the Great Ones, when she goes.

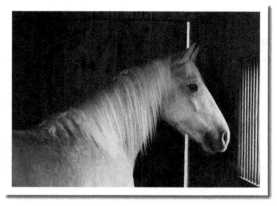

Left at Home

Beartown Mountain Bugaboo

I ask Mason if he would like to come along to Beartown State Park with me. He would remain on foot while I ride, but I feel like his presence would give me more confidence in this new terrain. Even though I would navigate the bridle paths solo, we would each have a cell phone and a park map, as well as a little adventure.

Mason agrees and gets his camera equipment. We take Blue Hill Road to the Beartown entrance, and once unloaded, I tell him that I'll probably be back in two hours or so, around 1:00 P.M. Peanut, unnerved by the flapping flags by the lake front, the strange planters, picnic tables, and elevated barbeques, is eager to get out of there. Bali is with us, and I think that gives Peanut some reassurance. My dog at least is another creature—*creature comfort*.

The trail is rough with lots of branches to break, clearing the way for the next happy trail rider. I pass a couple of middle-aged women with their two wee dogs. "We're heading back," they tell me. "This isn't a very nice trail."

Nice enough, I think, following the red arrows that are tacked to trees at every turn, though I find myself losing my way soon enough and wonder about turning around before it's too late, but my father's favorite motto was "*We never go back,*" so I push on, asking myself, "Where in the hell am I?"

Following the park assistant's advice, I take Wildcat Trail—*are there wildcats here?* And come to think of it, this place is also called Beartown! But off we go for about seven miles before the trail loops back. I'm well on my way to nowhere. Peanut is behaving beautifully, yet I am already conscious of our agreed upon meeting-up time. When riding, it's nice not to have to keep to a schedule. I check my cell phone, and it gives that warning beep that signals I am almost out of power. *Oh Boy.* So I turn it off, hoping to save at least thirty seconds to check in with Mason and tell him that I am probably lost.

I have the park map tucked in my pocket, but when I pull it out, I can't tell which way is up or down. Besides that, I can't really read the map without my glasses. But I figure I must be going in the right direction when we finally cross a road and the little red arrows—*like Hansel and Gretel's breadcrumbs*—lead me into the forest on the other side.

We should begin to head back toward the pond now—I have already been out for over two hours. I, at least, have my bottle of water tucked into my saddle pack, and I keep taking swigs. The woods are lovely. I am not afraid. I'm just glad I had eggs for breakfast.

We pass several woodsy marshes and move on through a tall pine forest of seemingly naked trees that go up and up and so do we, climbing, bending, wandering aimlessly—all of it lovely with bird song, and though it is warm, it is not stifling. My flannel shirt is handy. The pockets hold my cell phone, Chap Stick, gum, and tissue. I check to see if I have reception out here, and when I turn the phone back on, it makes that miserable little melody that indicates my cell phone is now dead. I eat the yoghurt I have in my saddle pack—lunch on the run. *Nervous?* Nah. I just have punctuality anxiety, and don't want to be inconsiderately late.

There are plenty of fallen trees to cross and several mucky passes where there are feeble wooden footbridges, not meant for the equestrian, surely. At one point, I dismount and lead Peanut over the mud so that he won't sink any deeper. I believe he is getting tired, but so am I and so is my dog. I wonder if Mason is having any fun, or is he looking at his watch wishing he had heard me yell—*"Pack a lunch."* I eat cherries from their ziplock baggie and am glad that I brought something to snack on.

The two middle-aged women made the right decision. I have no idea where I am or how long it will take to get back, so when I see a gravel road running parallel to the forest path, I decide to let it lead me onward. We canter a ways uphill. Peanut stumbles and goes down on one knee but quickly recovers. Still, what if he had gone lame?

Finally the gravel ends at a cement road, and I am now pretty well turned around. There is not a single road sign to show me the right direction. If this were Italy, there would be arrows pointing me to Florence from fifty miles away. I make a decision with total assurance and take a right on the paved road and ride in the wrong direction. Peanut has never ridden on pavement before in his life, with the exception of crossing a road from one field to the next. I worry that pushing him on this pavement might make him sore.

Finally, a car approaches. I wave it down by riding down the middle of the road. They have to stop, and they do. The couple is very friendly. I ask them where this road goes, and they say Route 102, toward Lee. *Whoops.* "Do you know where Benedict Pond is?" I ask, and luckily they have a GPS. At least someone is well equipped. Now they can assure me, beyond a shadow of a doubt, that all I have to do is turn around and ride another eight miles back on the pavement!

"Do you think I could use your cell phone?" I ask. "Mine is dead." But there is still no reception. So I ask them to do me a favor—"If you see a handsome man with a camera near a horse trailer in the second parking lot, could you tell him I'm on my way?"

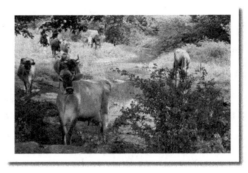

Cows by Alford Brook

Wilcox Farm

Yesterday, I took West Road through Alford, and when I passed the Wilcox Farm, I saw Ray Senior riding his lawnmower tractor and stopped to introduce myself. I had never heard back from Ray Junior about the possibility of riding in their valley, but the old man, almost ninety-four, thought it would be fine.

So today, Elizabeth and I head back to the Wilcox Farm, parking the trailer on the grass just beyond the barn where they are loading hay bales into the upper loft—quite a commotion. The horses skirt around this activity. Then, we head down the dirt road past a lot of suspicious farm machinery that the horses are loath to pass, but we push them forward and enter the genuine splendor of the valley.

At the first gate near the Alford Brook, I dismount, and a herd of cows starts heading our way. I want to get through, close the gate, and remount before they surround us. The odd thing about eastern cows is that they are so curious, expecting to be fed, whereas western cattle always leave you alone or head in the other direction.

There are lovely, tall trees by the little brook. It is so idyllic. We could be in the English countryside. The big fields are freshly mown to perfection. We canter up the rolling hill to the top corner then head through the woods into an upper area where Ray Junior is now busy baling. The machine he rides is whisking hay into tidy rows, and we are careful not to get in his way.

Approaching East Road, we hear a lone horse whinnying, and our horses respond as if anxious for him. I wonder if he is saying something they can understand—*Come rescue me. I'm lonely here!*

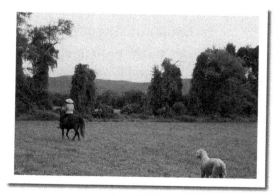

Open Fields

"I used to ride with my son here," I tell Elizabeth. "One time we were galloping along and Ayler's pony came to an abrupt halt, putting her head down. Ayler did a perfect somersault over her neck and landed on his feet." Star also had the habit of pawing water when we crossed a stream, which often meant that she was about to lie down, saddle, pad, rider, and all. Ayler came to realize that he had to kick her forward through the water before she got the idea for a swim in her mischievous head.

Back at the truck, I get out my basket to collect fresh corn. I tell Ray Senior that I'm going to make him some fresh corn chowder.

Sitting out on our deck, I shuck the husks, then steam the tender white ears of corn and scrape the kernels off. Boiling the bare cobs in chicken broth with carrots and onions creates a sweeter stock.

When I drive my container back over to the farm, Ray Senior is sitting out on the porch by himself, holding a fly swatter. He knocks the arm of his rocking chair with his cane. "Come sit down with me," he says. I ask him if he thinks the torn wicker seat will hold me. He says he wants to have it repaired, but he doesn't know if anyone does cane work anymore, and if someone did, it would cost a fortune. We talk about my mother-in-law, Emily Rose, who is now one-hundred-and-one. Not too many old-timers left from their generation, but Ray is sharp and knows the names and history of everyone around here.

"My father bought this farm when I was just five years old," he claims. "It was a dirt road then, but we didn't mind when it became macadam because moving a wagon and team of horses through spring mud was terrible work. It took all day to get to town." Now, it takes about fifteen minutes.

Paul, a farmhand, and Ray Junior have finished baling hay, and two truckloads go by to be stored in a back barn. I will need to buy some for winter. Paul joins us and says how he is planning on separating out cream from his milk later this afternoon. That will be a good addition to their chowder. I can hear a little calf bawling, and Paul says it is because the calves were just separated from their mothers last night. "They're missing the teat," he explains, but that's why fresh cream will soon be available.

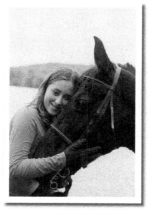

Avia

Too Much for Marcello

My goddaughter, Avia Rose Stanton, is going to ride with me this morning. I decide to bring both dogs, as I don't think we'll be out for long, but soon the temperature rises and so does the humidity. The dogs' coats are heavy, ready for grooming. Again, I am afraid a two-hour ride might be too much for Marcello, but both dogs are eager to go. They jump in the truck and then happily follow us through the fields.

We ride down to Phillip's Road, which we used to call "the dump road" and go back into a wilder area. The access to this field is chained off, but we go around through the tall weeds and ride all the way down to Marsh Pond. It is not farmland here, like most of Baldwin Hill, but hilly and rough. The views of Mount Washington are remarkable. The marsh itself is a wonderful habitat and would be a great place to go canoeing.

Back on the dump road, we take a little path that heads into the forest. It winds through acres of deep woods. We have trouble finding our way back to the open fields but finally see light ahead. As we wander back to the trailer, poor Marcello seems especially tired, and as soon as we get close, he lies down, pancake style, in the middle of the road, panting. I give him water from my bottle, pouring it down his throat. Marcello is still flat-out when a truck from the Turner Farm stops, wanting to get by. I am worried that Cello might be experiencing heat stroke. Did I push him too far? Maybe, these summer rides are too much for him now. Farmer Turner is patient while I pull Marcello out of the way and get him into the truck where I keep giving him big gulps of water. Then, we're off to a full recovery.

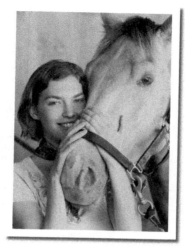

AZ and Peanut

Red Umbrella

"Do you have a waterproof jacket?" I ask my young friend, Arizona Muse. After all, the English would never go riding if they had to wait for sunshine. It's not bad going out in a light rain. We're not going to melt. My riding pants are soon damp, but I'm not uncomfortable. We move along on solid footing down by Long Pond, and Barranca gets into the smoothest fast walk I've ever experienced. All is fine until the horses spot Mr. Lawrence Barbieri's huge red umbrella. He is also out for a stroll, passing the lily-pad pond, and headed our way. The horses want nothing to do with him or his oversized red umbrella. I signal to Arizona that we should move uphill and wait until he passes. Once he has gone by, we follow him back along the same pond-side trail, riding through a fine mist. The curious thing is, the horses don't seem to mind the red umbrella when they know they are headed home.

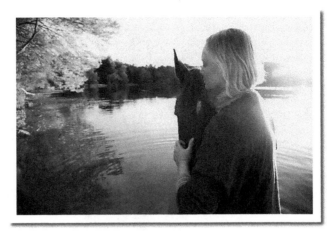

By the Pond

Back to Beartown

Elizabeth has been hankering to go to Beartown, and this Saturday seems like the perfect day—warm, glittery, clear air without a bug in sight. We caravan over to Benedict Pond with Mason and Elizabeth following in their cars. Near the upper parking lot, children are lolling about on their camp beds, having spent the night outside. They are eager to pat the horses.

Today, I want to ride near the pond on the footpath, until we meet up with the equestrian trail, but I forgot how difficult this path can be for horses. There are fallen trees blocking our way, treacherous slabs of rock to skate over, rough roots and marshy bogs with narrow foot bridges, which we will have to bypass.

Elizabeth is beginning to wonder if she is on an Outward Bound challenge, but I assure her that the trail up ahead is lovely. "It can't be far," I say, and at last, we find it, cheering out loud for the nice open space it provides.

While still encased in the overhang of late summer trees, with little peeks of the pond down below, we enjoy a canter or two until we come to a wooden footbridge. Barranca refuses to cross at first but finally gives in. Then, away we go, heading down an even more bucolic lane—we could be in Thomas Hardy country.

In another hundred yards, we see something that amazes us—an inkblack bear cub *galumphing* across the trail. "Where there's a cub, there's usually a sow," but we are thrilled at having seen this piece of raw animated nature out here in the middle of the day. We decide to ride on by. "*I heard that bears hate opera!*" I sing out loud, but the little one has disappeared into the forest with its bright rippling hide, glistening like a blackberry, possibly out searching for just that.

We decide to head back to a luncheon spot near the pond, finding a large, flat stone that faces the water. Just as we are settling down, a Golden Retriever joins us. He splashes into the water and lurches back up onto my stone platform to drench my riding breeches. I am not really bothered and give him some chicken from my sandwich. After that, he is a devoted friend.

Once back at the trailer, we unsaddle the horses. Then I hop back on Barranca, telling Elizabeth how I rode bareback in the Mississippi Rodeo years ago in a musical chair contest. "I was riding a big white horse named Washtub," I say. I remember that it was drizzling, and I made quite a scene sliding around in the mud, having to mount and dismount without the help of a saddle. I almost made it to the final round, but then I tied with an older guy, and we had to flip a coin. He won. Still, when I rode on out of the arena, I received a standing ovation and felt like I had triumphed.

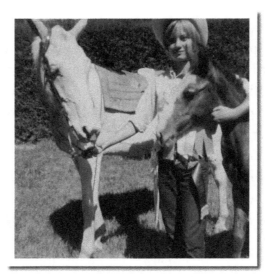

Mississippi

One of the most exciting experiences of my childhood was getting my Rough Rider badge at the Teton Valley Ranch Camp. You had to be able to rope your own horse, saddle him up, and cry out, "Ready to Ride, *Sir*," in a matter of minutes. Then we were off, plunging through rivers, galloping up steep terrain. We had to take off our saddles and ride bareback through a drainage ditch that ended up in a muddy sink hole. Here, we tied up our mounts, and the counselors proceeded to pass live snakes from hand to hand. This part almost did me in. We were then blindfolded and told that they were going to "milk" the snakes into our mouths (though they squirted lemon juice instead) before letting the snakes go in the muddy water. A wild mud-fight began that left us covered from head to toe. Only then did we ride back through camp at a gallop. *Quite an initiation!*

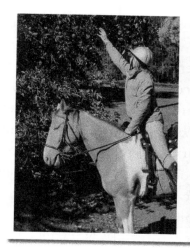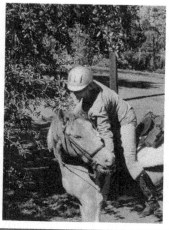

Picking / Feeding

Apple Chapel

This has been one hell of a year for apples! Or perhaps, I should say, *heavenly*. Every single tree is bearing an abundance of fruit. They spill all over the field with new ones down everyday. They hang in clumps on dipping limbs ready to be plucked, and believe me my horses know where they are. If one of my boys breaks free, he hightails it to the orchard to gorge on fallen apples.

I have been gathering apples for weeks now, first from Em's large, twin trees out in front of her house, and more recently from her new orchard. Though these are only adolescents, as trees go, they are producing some mature-looking, womanly apples, not unlike many overdeveloped teenage girls, ripe and ready to go before they are really grown-up.

I fill the golf cart's two wicker baskets and leave them in the tack room, which is always nice and cool. Then, I start to fill my market bags, some cardboard boxes, buckets, and coolers, as well as white plastic trash bags. I put boxes and cartons of apples in the basement, turning it into a makeshift root cellar, realizing that at some point I will need to cull through the lot of them and discard the rotting ones.

Today, I take my mother-in-law some elderflower jelly. Davina Muse, Em's most lovely caregiver, is intrigued and wants a taste as well. She tells me how her English parents kept their apples in a special apple-house with slotted drawers so that not one apple could touch another. That does seem wonderful, but I don't have anything like that. Maybe, I should store the apples in our little stone chapel.

"*The Apple Chapel,*" Davina agrees.

Em has finished her shepherd's pie and is now delving into the elderflower jelly—a pale golden color—and the taste is divine. Davina samples some, "Very subtle." She is a big fan of the elderberry bush and makes all sorts of medicinal concoctions from the fruit.

I am off to collect more apples, stopping at the one lone tree in the upper field. The horses haven't gotten to this one yet, and the limbs are laden with yellow fruit, ripe and unblemished. I begin to gather and quickly fill up my new containers. The horses are in for a very sweet winter.

I am beginning to wonder: *How many apples can a big horse munch if a big horse has access to apples?* I know there is a limit. I am already giving each horse about six apples a day, a couple at a time, slicing them up so that the smaller fruit doesn't get caught in the esophagus. I just hope Little Rose Chapel will protect these apples, keep them cool and safe. If not and they rot, I might take it personally, as if I were the fallen apple with a bad blemish. Please forgive me for being such a greedy gatherer. But maybe it's not so terrible to hoard such bounty when it's not for me but for my hungry horses.

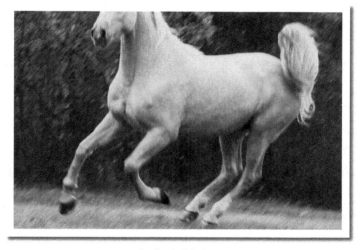

Rocket in Motion

Swarm

Barranca and Rocket are both saddled up, waiting in their stalls when my cousin Helen arrives from Colrain where she has a summer house. I am happy to go out in the late afternoon as the heat of the day is diminishing, and it is lovely riding through the forest into the golden late light. Rocket keeps breaking into a trot to keep up with Barranca but, Helen agrees, he has a wonderful canter.

Helen and I have been riding companions for as long as I can remember. Growing up together on Oconomowoc Lake, one year apart, we were like sisters. Sometimes, competition would flare up between us, and we would have a knockdown, drag-out fight over something as stupid as a plastic pad of fake butter, but for the most part we were daily companions.

Firstborn daughters, we both had difficult mothers, though Helen's mom fit in, for she was the daughter of my grandfather's roommate at Princeton and his best friend—Dr. Wilder Penfield, a renowned brain surgeon, while my mother's father, Mordecai Giffin Sheftall, worked on the railroad in the Deep South.

Aunt Priscilla was highly organized and had charts for chores that had to be completed before Helen could come out and play. Sometimes, wanting my cousin to be set free so we could head to the barn, I would come up into their loft apartment and help her sweep. Aunt Priscilla told me that if I couldn't do a job happily and nicely, it was best not to do it at all.

At other times, I was left waiting on the lawn while Helen had her enforced reading time after lunch. I had little interest in books at that age—there was far too much to do. I couldn't help her read, so I just had to wait, and then wait some more— then off we'd go to the family farm where we'd visit the old head gardener, Krietz. He was going blind, so we'd sneak one of his Chesterfield cigarettes while he was offering us butterscotch, the one kind of candy I didn't like.

Aunt Priscilla was hard on Helen, just as my mother was on me, but perhaps for different reasons. Helen's younger sister, Caroline, appeared to be the favorite—she was quite beautiful and did everything perfectly, while Helen and I were considered the black sheep of the family. I was amazed that Helen would dare steal a silver dollar from her mother's wallet. She got kicked out of school for smoking, and developed a reputation with a few "townie" guys. Helen was brazen enough to bring marijuana seeds back from Kenya on one of our family trips. She put the contraband in her camera case and planted the seeds in our grandmother's garden. One of Gramma's Garden Club ladies identified the plants. When Lyle Downs, the new gardener, was informed, he said he thought they were some sort of tomato plant (though he knew perfectly well what they were).

Even though Helen was one year younger, she was always more daring. She liked to initiate games of strip poker, which horrified me with my undeveloped body. But she was always comfortable in her skin. I didn't even like anyone watching me brush my teeth.

There aren't many people with whom you can share your whole childhood history, who have witnessed the upsets and family gatherings over the years. Together we shared our passion for horses. Our memory banks were full of similar information, including the songs that Gramma taught us, sung in rounds—"Make new friends, but keep the old, new are silver but the old are gold."

In the middle of the night we have a thunderstorm, but the morning is bright, windy, and clear. I am riding Peanut today, and Helen is riding Rocket. We unload on Baldwin Hill and pass through numerous fields, one yielding to the next. This hilltop land is so expansive and well-maintained. Mature trees stand between each section, serving as windbreaks in the winter.

"There's something nice about farmland up high on a hill, isn't there? You feel as if you're closer to the sky," Helen says. We spot a flock of Canada geese as we take a little path to the side where burrs stick to my pants and Peanut's blanket. I busy myself, plucking them off. Autumn is surely coming— as burrs stick and birds migrate.

Moving along the path, Peanut suddenly leans down, aggravated, and then seems frantic. Helen yells out, "Bees!" I turn and see Rocket dancing up and down as the bees swarm up all around us. I try to maneuver Peanut away from the path, out into the field, turning to see that Rocket is bucking and rearing. Helen doesn't know what to do. I jump down and yell at her, "*Get Off!*"

"I don't think I can!" she screams.

Rocket is going up on his rear legs, trying to get away. I rush over and grab his reins and tell her to bail—she does, hitting the ground with an audible thud. Then, I dash both horses out into the field. Helen comes after, huffing and puffing. I take off my flannel shirt and swing it around my head to discourage the last few lingering bees.

We lead the horses further away and wait to catch our breath before attempting to mount again. I decide to ride Rocket now, in case he is too worked up. The bees have disappeared and we are safe. Neither Helen nor I got stung, and Bali managed to stay away from the swarm altogether, unfazed by the attack.

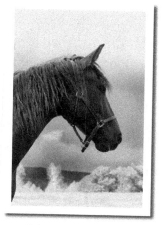

Calm before the Storm

Round Pond

Perhaps because of the solemnity of the day, September eleventh, the air seems particularly still, as blue and clear as it was nine years ago when the world was left in shock by the attacks on the World Trade Center.

I saddle up Barranca and decide to take him out alone, heading along the top of the ridge, planning to take a new path down toward Round Pond. Riding through the sarsaparillas, a tunnel of grey opens to a chartreuse splash at the end.

Soon, the new path disappears into unmarked woodland, but we continue bushwhacking along. No one has been down here in a long time, and there are lots of branches to break. We reach a treacherous slide of rocks, but with a little urging, Barranca makes it over. I keep expecting to spot a glimpse of the pond, but all I see is palomino-colored bracken, the magnificent forest dressed up in green and gold.

Finally, I spot a bit of blue through the leaves and know we are almost there. I feel a definite thrill, riding this new trail for the first time. I'm inside the moment, and Barranca is all fired up. When we hit the dirt road at water level, we canter to the end of the lake where there is a manmade dam. Standing there, looking out over the pond, I hear someone shooting a gun, target practice, getting ready for hunting season, no doubt, and it is disturbing. Guns, ammunition, explosions, crashes, towers collapsing—why is there so much destruction when peace can surround us?

By the time I get home, Barranca is covered with pine needles. As my feet hit the solid earth, I feel grounded, as if I have somehow absorbed my horse's sure-footedness and a powerful surge of energy moves through me, passing into my core.

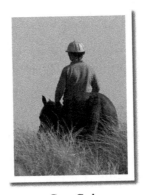

Cape Cod

Riding by the Sea

Saltwater Farm in Chatham, Massachusetts, is a funky little stable, but the horses are all in good shape. I will be riding a chestnut mare named Roxy. Vicci and her boyfriend load up all three horses, and we follow them over to the seashore.

It is a windy morning and quite a bit cooler, but the sun is shining and the horses are familiar with the sand and the sea. Today is the first legal day for riding on the beach so I lucked out. We take a trail on the land side of the dunes to warm the horses up and Roxy seems quite manageable.

Reaching the lighthouse at the end of the trail, we head over to the beach where Vicci tells me, "When the tide is out, you can ride all the way out on the sandbar to that buoy." But the tide is not radically in or out, just somewhere in between. She walks her horse into the lapping shallows, and I follow. The horses seem to enjoy the cooling effect of the water. Then, we ride back onto the hard-packed sand, and Vicci suggests a canter. I'm game. They say how Roxy has a nice, slow, plodding canter, but once we take off, it is more like a racing gallop. Not familiar with this horse, I'm a bit apprehensive—I don't know if she might shy or buck, but I lean forward, standing up slightly in my stirrups as she races the others. Finally, I rein her in, exhilarated to be riding by the sea.

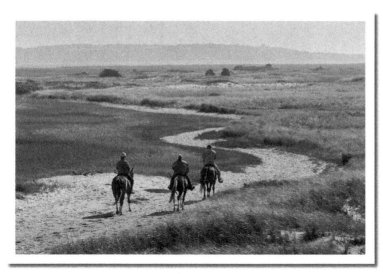

Dunes

For the next stretch, I suggest that I go ahead so that it doesn't turn into a contest of speed. At a slower pace, this mare is much more comfortable. I feel relaxed and confident now, but then we see a windsurfer up ahead. I am astounded when he leaps off a wave and soars into the air at least ten-feet high. The handheld sail is moving him along at about thirty miles per hour, and as we head back to our destination, it looks like he is shooting right at us—maybe he's thinking of coming into shore. We wave to alert him and steer the horses back towards the dunes. Isn't he looking? Or maybe he doesn't care about spooking three large horses. He continues to fly in our direction, and the horses are skittish, as well they should be! But then, he leaps into the air again and swings off in another direction.

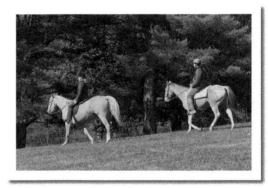

Daphne and Kevin

Columbus Day Weekend

My niece, Daphne, and her fiancé, Kevin Crowe, arrive on Saturday morning with their Springer Spaniel, Sawyer—a beautiful puppy with perfect, symmetrical markings on his face. Bali and Cello are eager to play with him, and he is ecstatic to have free run, splashing in the rock garden pool, exploring the horse pasture. In fact, he is quite entranced by the horses, as if he thinks they are enormous dogs.

After lunch, we put Sawyer in his crate and saddle up the horses. Daphne is a great rider. I know she can handle Rocket's little quirks, and Kevin surprises us by being very competent. I take them down to Long Pond to see the autumnal splendor reflected in the water, and then up we go to the top of the ridge, cantering through the pine forest. Daphne's long golden hair is held back in a ponytail, and she is relaxed in the saddle even though Rocket has already given a couple of bucks.

The next morning, Daphne and I ride alone together. She is happy to have Barranca today. I work with Peanut, who seems to have lost his natural four-beat gait—partly a problem of having so many different riders over the course of the summer. The euonymus is just beginning to turn a pale pink color, but soon the low-growing bushes will dazzle these woods with candy-apple red.

Daphne is a reserved young woman with amazing intellect, happily in love with her fiancé, Kevin. She tells me that she knew she would marry him when he sat with Grandma on the porch one afternoon, reading *Life's Little Instruction Book* out loud to her, with Grandma commenting all along the way. "I thought, if he's patient enough for that activity, he'll be able to put up with me."

Daphne is also a "family planner." I have told her how that can be a thankless task. Still, we seem to persist in being the Little Red Hens with a bunch of Chicken Littles around us.

Always one of Grandma's favorites, I know Daphne had a very different experience of my mother than I did. When Mom was descending into Alzheimer's, she called Grandma every day to check on her.

"You know growing up," Daphne admitted, "I hated anything that was a salad sandwich...chicken salad, tuna salad, ham salad, egg salad...but those were Grandma's favorites, so I would DESPERATELY try to avoid having lunch with her out at the lake. Eventually, I learned to negotiate for a hot dog before accepting an invitation."

Daphne recalled how much Grandma loved to lie out on her plastic white and yellow chaise in the garden of Broadoaks, hiking up her housedress to tan her legs, how she would swim every afternoon along the lakeshore in her rubber cap and old-fashioned suit, then rest on the raft or dock. "And boy did she love those Kiltie milkshakes!"

"And chocolate," I added. "She was crazy for chocolate."

At one of our big Thanksgivings dinners in Patagonia, she hoarded all the chocolates that were being passed out by our Swiss friends—guarding them in her lap like a small child before gobbling them up.

"I remember Grandma always doing her nails," Daphne said. At the end of her life it became an obsession. "And her buzzing around in that golf cart. She really loved that golf cart."

One week when Grandma was in town, the grandchildren found the hidden key in a dresser drawer and took the golf cart for a spin. They ended up crashing it into a tree, denting the fender. Though they had the damage repaired, Grandma knew there was something different. "This cart doesn't drive like it used to."

Daphne used to work in Grandma's garden every afternoon, picking fresh vegetables with her for dinner. "One day, Abigail and I decided to be industrious, and we had a vegetable stand out by Sawyer Road." All went well until Grandma returned and saw them hawking her produce by the side of the road without having asked permission!

But Daphne's favorite part of the summer week was Sunday evening, sitting with Grandma and Popi out on the porch, while they watched 60 Minutes, their favorite show. They would each enjoy a glass of white wine and Daphne would create a cheese plate for everyone to enjoy. "I felt so loved and supported by both of them," she said wistfully.

I think of how lucky we were to have a summer place that had been in the family for generations. Now my cousins were putting together a scrapbook of all the horses from the family farm, with photographs dating back to our grandparents day: Stories of the mischievous Bunko; Busytown with his rocking horse canter; Eagle, the horse Gramma bought for me, shipping him all the way home from Montana; Sharif, my grandfather's prize-winning jumper; the ponies—Lady and Texas; and who could forget that chestnut, Frisky, the nasty mare who would pin her ears back and chase us across the pasture.

"Do you remember how Grandma used to wear those wonderful Mexican house dresses all around the house during the summer? Now my Mom is wearing those exact same dresses around Broadoaks!"

Daphne's parents purchased the family home from Cia and me, and they have done extensive renovations. Daphne pitched in every weekend she was there, doing endless chores without complaint.

There were stories that the house was haunted—Daphne and her cousin had seen an apparition moving through the dining room, and others had heard furniture shoved around at night. Years ago, my sister had experienced disturbing spirits in her third floor bedroom, and it had been pivotal in her conversion to Christianity. You couldn't pay me to sleep alone in that house, but the ghost never bothered my mother.

Daphne recalled Grandma's visits to their ranch in Montana and how she loved nothing more than to go float-boating down the Madison River. "I'm not sure if she did any fishing, but she loved floating downriver, taking in the beautiful scenery."

During Daphne's last visit to see Grandma in Arizona, she was swimming in the pool while Grandma sat out on the deck watching her. "When I climbed out of the pool, Grandma commented, 'You have very nice legs...just so you know...you got those from me!'" We had to laugh over that one.

"I remember when Grandma called me one evening to tell me that she had just been diagnosed with Alzheimer's," Daphne recalled, not laughing now, serious, sad. I could tell that she missed her Grandma. "I was living in New York at the time and had just gotten home from work. She was so upset, crying on the phone. She said that she wanted to be the one to let me know. She told me that she loved me, and she wanted to be sure to tell me how much she loved me before she might not remember anymore.

"But mainly I remember how happy Grandma and Popi were most of the time, especially when they were just by themselves. They were always holding hands, or he'd have his arm around her shoulder. On my visits to Arizona I would find them lying in bed together, holding hands, talking and laughing. I think they really loved each other."

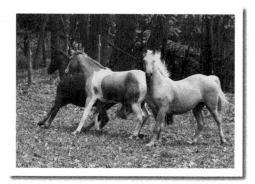

In the Paddock

Euonymus Woods

There are only a couple of more weeks before Peanut is shipped out West. I hope the transition is not too hard on him. At least he won't have to suffer a cold Berkshire winter with his thin skin. But now I am beginning to wonder why I have not heard from the horse transport people.

I go online and am horrified when I discover a string of testaments from people who claim *Cornerstone Equine Transport* ripped them off, scam artists! I have already sent off a certified check for over $600, half-payment, but now when I try to find the Cornerstone website, it no longer exists. I try calling their toll-free number and leave messages on all four bogus extensions, wondering if anyone will ever get back to me.

After a frantic morning of phone calls, trying to arrange for another driver, I am beside myself, scattered and distracted, trying to get ready for my upcoming trip to India. Putting one's faith and trust in some unknown hauler is a big deal when it comes to the health and safety of a precious animal. I feel vulnerable, ripped off, but mostly angry at myself for being so careless—why did I not get references? What I really need right now is a good, long ride to regain my equilibrium.

Barranca seems slowed by his thickening coat, but he is still my willing boy. As we ride into the euonymus woods, the whole lower portion of the forest is now painted a bright pink-red that spreads over the woodland floor like a luxurious comforter.

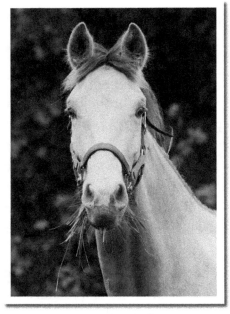

What Did I Do?

Bliss on Barranca

Indian summer must be the most beautiful time of year— delightful to have this humid warmth with the rust and burnt-gold leaves still waving. Everything is so perfect on this seventy-degree day it makes me want to stall time and stay right here, suspended.

I want to enjoy these last few rides on Barranca alone, taking in the fairytale spectacle of the cherry-colored woods, a cardinal flitting through the burst-open bittersweet. Suddenly, up ahead, the most magnificent buck springs across the trail, disappearing into the forest.

Barranca seems to walk gingerly, as if knowing that the leaf-covered paths could hide treacherous roots and potholes. He is taking his time, picking his way as we head down to the Alford Road. Cutting across the pavement into the woods, we try to find a new route over to the brook, but Barranca trips on a hidden strand of barbed wire and panics. "*Whoa,*" I say, hopping off to hold the wire down with my boot, easing his hoof back over it.

I wonder if he has memories of the barbed wire accident that cut him up before I bought him. Such traumas lodge in the cellular memory, but luckily that memory doesn't overwhelm him. He is such a steady horse. I believe he trusts me as much as I do him.

Going through a narrow opening into the lower fields, I see that the goldenrod has aged from a greenish-blond to grayish fuzz. There is an abundance of berries—little white ones pop on their frail grey stems all along the field, and red berries dangle like miniature Tic-Tacs. A crab apple tree is laden with fruit that almost resembles tiny plums. I take a nibble, and it is sour, not for human consummation. Some of the maples are still fully clothed in vibrant gold while others have been stripped bare.

Light glazes the wings of a raven flying off across the field as we canter on the curving imprint of a tractor track. Big piles of firewood are seasoning by the hedgerow. I know cold weather is coming and that this is but a brief respite. We are in that perfect moment of appreciated warmth before autumn turns harsh and punishing. The milkweed is opening, and I snatch a pod and let the parachute wishes cascade behind me—such balmy air, such glorious colors.

As we enter the woods behind Peck's Pick Farm, a sifting of pale yellow leaves twirls around us. We seem suspended in time.

Why does Barranca feel like the perfect partner? Why does he seem to understand me, almost without direction? If there is such a thing as an "old soul" in an animal, he surely has one. How lucky I am to have found this horse.

At home, I bring out two big pails of warm water and wash him down with a sea sponge, shampooing his mane and tail, using Cowboy Magic conditioner to untangle his locks. My two little mischief makers look over the fence as if wondering—"Why is *he* getting so much attention while the two of us have to stay behind the rails?"

Because, I think, you are naughty boys who have been breaking out of your pasture—you are having an Equine Time Out!

As I wash Barranca's legs, I see that some of the milkweed fluff has stuck under his foreleg—a sign of good luck for my best boy. How I will miss him, but I don't want him to suffer that long haul twice a year. I turn him out into the upper field to graze, watching the dark shine of his skin as it dries in the afternoon sun.

INDIA

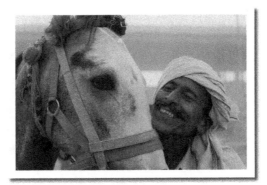

Halfway around the World

Varanasi Carriage Ride

On our first evening in Varanasi, we walk through the teeming market streets down to the crowded *ghats* where temples, shrines, and palaces loom like fantastic sandcastles from ancient times. The Ganges moves slowly under a darkening sky as seven Brahmin priests in peach-colored satin perform the evening ceremony, swinging powerful incense to the sound of tabla drums. Then, the long walk back, stepping over garbage and cow pies, spotting one big bull lounging on the floor of a local shop as if it was his normal, nocturnal resting place.

The people of Varanasi seem to have a certain glow about them. Perhaps this stems from daily lives steeped in spiritual practice and devotions. But how can any religion keep track of over a million gods? Does that simply mean that almost everything earthly is permeated by the spiritual realm?

We wake at five in the morning to get back to the Ganges for a sunrise boat tour, and in the morning light, we are more aware of the ash-grey pollution of the river. Cremations are blazing away on the riverbanks, and off to the right, the bloated body of a dead goat makes Ayler gag. He turns his attention to his little ghee candle and sets it afloat in a marigold laden boat.

When I think about my mother's cremation in Wisconsin, I realize how different death is in our culture. Soon after her passing, my mother's body was zipped into a black plastic bag and whisked away to be held in cold storage. As is typical in America, no one attended to her body. No one was there for her cremation. A few days later, her remains, ground to a fine grey powder, were placed in a tidy box.

Mom wanted her ashes spread on the desert in Arizona. I would have to transport them. My sister brought a bag of "Mom" to the Lake Club, plunking them down on the dinner table. Our brother David was appalled—"You two and those ashes! Now you see why your brothers have a problem with their sisters!"

We were clearly four different individuals, but the older you get the more you becomes yourself, as if the sauce of personality is reduced, intensified. But we were still a family, like it or not. We were still the children of Margaret and George, no matter what we felt they had or hadn't given to us. Now it was our turn to stop the blaming, and turn to ourselves, and try to make the best of it. One has to accept one's own flaws in order to find forgiveness. Now it was our turn. Next, it would be theirs—our children, grandchildren, down through the progressing years that were passing more quickly than we believed possible.

In India, multiple lifetimes are ever-on-going. Waiting for the sun to make its appearance through the smog, the devout are taking their purification baths, washing away sins and bad karma, modestly changing out of wet clothes by pulling dry ones over their heads.

We work our way back through the claustrophobic sensory overload, trying to avoid the *bindi* sellers and postcard hawkers who are far more tenacious and annoying than any beggar. Traveling in India, I am reminded of what people did *not* tell me about childbirth, avoiding any accounts of discomfort or pain, only focusing on the joys of motherhood. Similarly, I feel that friends who have told me of their travels in India only mentioned the amazing colors, the fabulous markets, the great deals, and rarely the extreme pollution or the distressing poverty, the chaos of the roads where it is truly survival of the fastest.

After lunch, my traveling companion, Lizbeth Marano, and I explore the hotel gardens and come upon a skinny, little man leading a white, Rajasthani stallion with big black balls. The horse has the typical Marwari ears that curve inward. He seems to be quite docile, following this man about without lead rope or halter.

Neemsha is the horse-trainer for the Palace Hotel next door to our rather mediocre abode. The abutting garden looks like a very grand, serene place, just beyond the guarded gates. We are not allowed to pass into this highly exclusive property, once home to the King of Benaras. We want to see the palace stables, and the guard suggests that we check with the concierge at our hotel. Neemsha is currently busy hooking up the stallion to an antique black carriage. Wouldn't it be fun to get a ride?

We learn that Neemsha is one in a long line of horse trainers—his father and grandfather before him had been the horsemen of the palace. This little man with bad teeth and shining eyes plays polo and races and trains. "I can do anything with horses," he tells us.

At the hotel desk, I ask the concierge if we can get a tour of the palace stable nextdoor. "I am writing a book about riding," I tell her, and that does the trick. Within minutes, Neemsha returns in a long, clean white shirt and crimson turban, instantly transformed, ready to give us a tour right from the front of our hotel. Lizbeth and I both climb into the back of the carriage, and off we go through the now open gate. As we cover the grounds on a soft dirt path that circles the gardens, our driver points out various trees and plants along the way—fragrant jasmine and formal roses. Peacocks roam, and palm trees sway.

Neemsha then suggests that I climb up front into the driver's seat and take the reins, calling out "*Chella!*" (*let's go*) to his stallion. The horse begins to pace and then breaks into a canter. Still, he is not difficult to hold. We pull up beneath the *porte cochere* of the Palace Hotel where we are invited to enter. As we cross the marble entryway, there seem to be more servants in traditional attire than hotel guests.

You can arrange to have a private dinner for two on the massive expanse of lawn and watch your own private fireworks display. But with over four-hundred festivals a year in Varanasi, it hardly seems necessary to add to the *diwali* excitement where the cacophony of explosions is enough to set off anyone's startle response. The Varanasians appear to have a bubbling sense of joy, harmony, and balance, coupled with amazing immune systems, able to survive and flourish amidst the unsanitary conditions.

Driven back to our lesser hotel in this regal antique carriage, the white stallion imperiously takes a big dump at the front door as we jump out and tip our smiling driver.

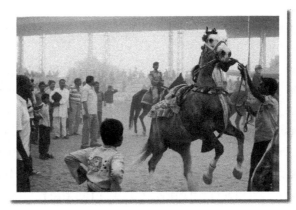

The Stadium

Pushkar Camel and Cattle Fair

Camels and fabulous horses are spread out amongst this primitive tent city, covering acres and acres of rolling pasture. We meander through a herd of water buffalo with their low-moaning calls, until we come to the horses, many of them tethered by all four feet so they can't kick out. Most of the horses look well cared for, with the exception of the occasional emaciated mare. There are a lot of young Marwaris for sale, often standing by their mothers' side. Camel-cart taxis pass us everywhere, and feral gypsy children try to get money from us, cursing us when we do not produce a coin—*unnerving*.

We finally come upon the big arena where a few men are trying out horses on thick, cloth pads set very far back, making their horses go into high-speed running walks, at least as fast as a flat-out gallop. The riders sit perfectly still. This four-beat *revaal* gait is incredibly smooth, even at this speed.

One magnificent pinto stallion is the most remarkable creature, very high strung, not used to all this commotion, but his handler is managing him somehow. Undoubtedly there are plenty of mares in heat in the surrounding area, and it must be making him crazy.

We buy several colorful cotton halters with dangling strips and pom-pom top-knots, haggling over the price of each item. But carrying a plastic bag marks me for other people hawking stuff. These young men persist, trying to bargain with me over something I clearly don't want. I am forced to be rude—"NO, I wouldn't want that even if you gave it to me!"

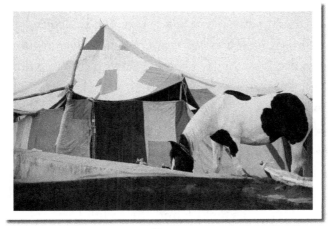

Pinto

Excited about our trail ride on the following morning, we walk back to Camp Bliss and relax before dinner. The dining tent is lovely, made out of a warm amber-colored Indian print material. The food is all vegetarian, delicious, but there is no alcohol allowed in the holy city of Pushkar. I could use a glass of wine.

Tiny lights are strung all over the gooseberry trees, which makes the place especially magical at night. Two comfortable canvas lounge chairs are placed outside of each sleeping tent. You can sit and listen to the evening drumming and watch the nightly entertainment of dancers, fire eaters, and jugglers who perform around the bonfire. We go to bed early, all set to rise for our ride, so long in the planning.

The equestrian tent camp, ten minutes away, is a rather miserable setup compared to the relative luxuries we have been enjoying at Camp Bliss. The horses are tethered out in individual spots, and I am curious to know which horse I will get. They all seem relatively small and thin. I just hope there is a good saddle left for me as all the other riders arrived the afternoon before and they have already gotten their horses and tack and taken a preparatory ride. We sit around a grubby, bare table with a few other women—mostly Germans—one of whom asks in a heavy accent, "Do you like to gallop?"

"Well, sometimes," I respond.

"*Goot*," she says, "then you are accepted."

There is one pleasant, young woman who is going to ride the owner's horse that morning, because the mount she'd originally been given was not appropriate for her. I wonder if my scrawny little mare, Angelie, will be comfortable, for she is as narrow as a skiff, and the saddle I receive is much too small. The metal rim embedded in the low cantle hits me at my coccyx, and while this does not seem to be a problem at first, it soon becomes painful. I try to remedy the problem by lengthening my stirrups, which could be a mistake.

Red ribbons are tied to most of the mares' tails, indicating they are kickers. I am told that Angelie is a "lead horse" and very fast despite her size. The leader of the morning ride is a handsome twenty-nine-year-old named Manu.

We go out into the desert where the landscape is strangely similar to Arizona, but very hot and humid. The trail we take is deep with soft, golden-brown earth. At least if anyone falls, they will be received by fortunate footing. But all of the horses seem to ride together in a clump, and while Manu keeps waving me back, indicating that I should stay away from his mare, I soon find that my horse has a very tough mouth and is extremely difficult to restrain. Undoubtedly, she has had so many riders pulling on her, trying to stop her from racing, that she has become unresponsive. Even while walking, the iron-rimmed cantle is jamming into me as Angelie bounces up and down, prancing sideways, wanting to go. I don't want to be a complainer, but the stirrup leathers are pinching the insides of my knees and it's beginning to seriously hurt. But this discomfort is nothing compared to what I feel once Manu suddenly gives the signal to *GO!* Then, the whole tight pack lights out at a dead-bolt run.

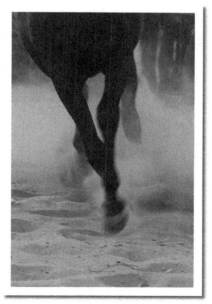

Desert Dust

Trying to hold my horse back from ramming into his, Angelie goes into a very choppy gait that makes me bounce in the saddle so that the stirrup leathers, snapping open and shut, are cutting into me like razors. We take several turns at full speed, and she almost slips. If she falls—I think—I will get trampled by the horses flying so close behind. I cannot believe the pace we are going with little preparation for this.

I worry about Lizbeth, who is somewhere toward the back of the pack. She must be riding in a cloud of dust, unable to breathe. Once we stop for a moment, before another burst of speed, some of the other riders request that we change order so that they can ride farther up front, out of the dust. *I'll change places with you, I think, if you'll trade horse and saddle!*

I wonder if I can ride like this for days. It feels as if there is nothing between my legs. When I mention the stirrup leathers, Manu seems unconcerned. We soon take off on another high speed tear. I try to relax, but the stirrup leathers are really eating into me. When we stop, I turn toward the back of the group and ride up to Lizbeth, saying in a whisper, "I think we should cancel."

"I'm so glad to hear you say that," she exclaims. "I was definitely going to drop out, and I was wondering what I would do, as I figured you'd just plow ahead."

"I've never been so uncomfortable on a horse in my life," I respond. "I feel like we might get seriously injured. It's just not worth it."

"Plus, it's not good for the horses," Lizbeth adds, "Flat out racing, everyone out of control." Lizbeth is a terrific rider who has been in dressage training for fifteen years. She recently imported a fabulous young Andalusian from Seville, Spain. Her final words on the subject of this ride—"*I am so out of here!*"

We both agree that we should call our travel agent, and try to do something else.

On returning to the disgusting tent-camp bathroom, I look at the inside of my legs and see that I am covered in raw, bruised marks. If I were to continue, I would probably end up bleeding.

I think about my tendency to always "plow ahead." I guess that had always been my way, to keep on going, to overachieve, to try and be the fastest and the best, partly my temperament and partly the way I was brought up. "I don't care what you do," my father once told me, "as long as you are number one." That was a heavy requirement to put on a small child.

We were expected to be self-reliant, independent, resilient in the face of torment, getting back in the saddle after being knocked off. Our father would lead across whitewater, down muddy embankments, even down the middle of railroad tracks, as if our uneasiness was titillating for him.

Once Popi even went so far as to spray bug repellent in the face of Cia's horse while she was holding baby Abigail. The horse reared and Abigail fell. I'm sure he felt remorse, but why was he being so careless?

My father often put me in uncomfortable situations—riding into a bull pasture with a bull whip in hand while I rode my pony. That created anxiety in me, an anxiety that is still beginning to surface, as I try to control situations so that I won't be late or panicked, having a somewhat compulsive need for daily ritual, becoming more reliant on habit.

My friends think of me as a fearless rider, but that is no longer true. As a child, one goes along with the program, rarely questioning, but now as an adult, I can weigh the risks and say, "No, I do not want to do this."

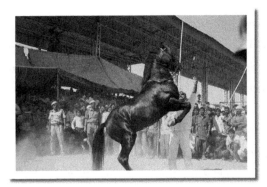

Dancing Stallion

We are both relieved to catch a jeep ride back to Camp Bliss where we call our travel agent and alert him to our change of plans. He is very understanding and comes up with an alternate itinerary in a matter of hours.

After lunch, we take a camel-cart taxi back to the main arena where we meet up with a young man named "Shom." He offers to let us ride his two camels back to Camp Bliss in the dusky afternoon light for a small fee of 250 rupees each. From the height of the camels, we get a good view of a dancing stallion that is up on his hind legs, bouncing to the rhythm of the drums, surrounded by a dense crowd of onlookers.

As we work our way back toward our tent camp, we witness a mare being bred. One man holds her tail out of the way while the huge member of the stallion extends. A few plunges and it's over. *"Finito,"* I say, and one of the local men laughs, understanding my meaning.

We pass through the darkening tent city where desert people are huddled about their fires—smoke rising. I almost feel like I am back in biblical times. Most of the horses are now clothed with makeshift, sackcloth blankets to protect them from the cold—*same impulse, different budget.* The horses are now busy with their fodder, peacefully eating while shy yet sparkly children wave.

The camel saddle and camel pace is decidedly comfortable, moving me back and forth on my padded perch, a rocking gait that suits me after this morning's trauma. But getting down off a camel feels rather weird as you descend in a three-part motion, as if sitting on a collapsing crane. Back on solid earth, we make plans for Shom to come meet us the following morning so that we can ride through the encampment at sunrise.

Waking early, along with the local roosters, it is nice to be up before everybody else. At the agreed upon time, Shom is there at the gate with his two camels, and up we go, rocking backward and forward in ascension. Shom gives me the two strings that attach to "Johnson's" nose bridle—a strange piercing that works as a nose-bit. It's rather fun steering my camel with these scanty, makeshift reins, while Shom leads Lizbeth up ahead. I am glad to be enjoying this nice rocking gait—it is very soothing even when Shom gets our mounts to do their own unique, exaggerated form of trotting. We enter the fair grounds and head toward the dunes where most of the camels are traded.

Herds of loose camels are ushered along the hillsides. In the dim light, we ride up to the top of one of the dunes and look down over the huge expanse. Dismounting, we decide to have a cup of morning chai just as the sun appears, blushing over the entire scene.

One young camel lets out a terrible screaming wail, and Shom explains that it is receiving a nose piercing. It sounds excruciating. We then hear whining pipe music and drums down below—a huddle of men sit in a circle around a couple of baskets. Live cobras rise to the music.

So many of the camels have glamorous saddle sheets or trinket-laden covers, hennaed heads and shaved markings, anklets and pom-poms—the gaudier the better. I tell Shom that I want to buy "Baby Camel Johnson" some decorative necklaces as a way of honoring our guide. He raised this camel since it was just a few months old. No wonder he seems so tame. Shom tells me that I could buy my own camel—it would only cost about $500. I could come back each year and try it out. I imagine that if my father were here, he would be quick to buy a camel just to have something to talk about. "What are they?" *Camels.* "What are they like?" *Steady, plodding, loyal.*

Shom selects ten colorful necklaces for a mere 150 rupees—(43 rupees to a dollar, so this gift amounts to about $3.50). He ties them onto the camels' long necks, one after another, and the pretty cotton balls of purple, green, pink, and red make a nice effect. The sun is now up, and we want to head back to the arena to see the "camel dancing."

The performing camels lift their large, split, pancake hooves to the drumbeat. One camel lies down on its side so the trainer can stand on top of him, perhaps to show his dominance over the animal's willing submission. In another unnatural stunt, the camel kneels on its forelegs and crawls forward slowly.

Lizbeth and I begin to feel like we are getting too much sun. The dancing horse performance seems extreme, almost frenzied. It makes me think of the mazurka—squatting down and thrusting out the legs—which couldn't be easy or healthy for a horse. We decide it is time to stretch our own legs. Dismounting, we say goodbye to Shom and "Baby Camel Johnson," walking on back to the serenity of Camp Bliss.

Later that day, on our drive to Jodhpur, we stop to have an afternoon cup of chai. While we sit outside in our plastic chairs, waiting for the tea to arrive, our driver explains, "This might take a minute—they had to run out and milk their cow."

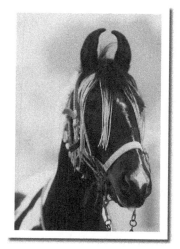

Marwari

Jodhpur and Rohet Garh

Sheer stone walls rise forty feet on either side of the entrance to the Raas Hotel, framing the illuminated levels of its amazing courtyard. High above, the massive Mehrangarh Fort rests on top of an impenetrable mountain. We are happy to have our creature comforts: luxurious bathrooms and king-size beds, balconies facing the lit-up fort where dangling lights hang over the ramparts. A small parade goes by on the street below, perhaps part of the bigger wedding party celebration going on in Jodhpur that evening.

There is a sad story behind this wedding. The young thirty-four-year-old prince, Shivraj Singh Ji, was in a serious polo accident five years ago and suffered a brain hemorrhage. He remained in a coma for three months, and while now partially recovered, his health is still severely compromised. He is soon to marry the twenty-two-year-old princess of Jaipur, and as in most royal Indian weddings, this will be an extravagant, colorful affair that will continue throughout the coming week.

The next day, we catch a taxi out to Rohet Garh, home of the Rajasthani gentleman, Sidharth Singh, who turned his family's fort into a lovely heritage hotel. As we drive from Jodhpur, the landscape appears unremarkable, flat, agricultural, but as we wind our way through the small village toward the entrance to the hotel, I am excited to see the stables straight ahead—the interior courtyard is padded with soft earth. There is a serene euphony of absence here, a relief to be far from the crowds and pollution and honking horns. We begin to feel very hopeful, sensing that at last we will have a good ride.

The six surrounding stalls of the stable all hold exquisite mares—one has a two-month-old colt with her—and the well-kept horses all turn inward to socialize as any female dormitory would do. When we meet our horseback riding guide, MD, this young trainer has such positive energy that again we are reassured. He tells me that I will be riding a stallion but emphasizes that Arbud is a very gentle horse. We can see that MD takes care with his horses, checking their legs and hocks and unshod feet before we go out.

The owner, Sidharth, greets us with the utmost hospitality, even though he is about to depart for Jaipur by train for the royal wedding. His Yellow Labrador is a bit of a surprise as it is the first fully bred dog I have seen in all of India. Our handsome host is eager for us to have a good ride. Sidharth and his staff have been working to bring the Marwari breed back into good repute, and from what we can tell, they are doing an excellent job. It is now 4:00 P.M. and we will go out into the fields for a couple hours. It is still warm but not too hot for the horses.

The Marwari were originally used as warrior horses. They are fearless and faithful with terrific stamina and endurance.

I wonder if it will be difficult to hold back my stallion, for as one driver told us—"What you need in India is a *good horn, good brakes, and good luck.*" But I would add—and a *good horse!*

Thankfully, my gentle, grey Marwari stallion has a very delicate mouth. The Pushkar ride damaged my self-confidence, but now it is quickly restored. The saddle fits perfectly, and I am grateful to get another try on a Marwari.

Lizbeth is given a rather spirited black mare who dances about, shying at motorbikes on the way out of town. MD is riding another black mare. Both of these young horses have only been in training for a matter of months. Soon, it becomes apparent that Lizbeth would do better on his horse so they exchange, and then she feels more at ease. Both mares seem more high-strung than my mount, but all of them are beautiful and have not been ruined by rough handling.

Rajasthan had a very good monsoon season this year, which broke a terrible drought. Now, the semi-arid landscape seems moist. The fields of mustard and millet have all been harvested, and the earth is still soft in places. MD is concerned that we have to pick the right place to canter so that the horses won't sink and strain their legs. It is good to be in the hands of a knowledgeable, responsible guide.

I keep my distance from the mares and ride behind as we head out alongside the fields on a soft, dirt road. Tractors and cattle carts pass us. A woman in a bright red sari carries a huge bundle of sticks on her head. Herds of goats graze with a young goatherder in attendance. All is calm and restful.

Lizbeth's horse is named Lakshmi, the goddess of good luck and wealth. She suits Lizbeth perfectly. My friend looks very well-balanced on this lovely mare whose neck is arched, collected. I notice that my horse, Arbud, has a perfect four-beat walking gait, and I take him ahead of the mares for a while, lifting my reins slightly and leaning back a bit to let him move out. But going first makes the two mares antsy, wanting to race, so I return to the rear. MD explains that the *revaal* gait—the running walk we witnessed in the arena at Pushkar (where the riders sat so far back, almost on the horses' rumps, sticking their feet way out in front of them)—is actually quite harmful to the animals. It puts all the rider's weight on the horse's haunches, making the horse lift his head, hollowing out his back. A consistent use of this gait often ruins a horse.

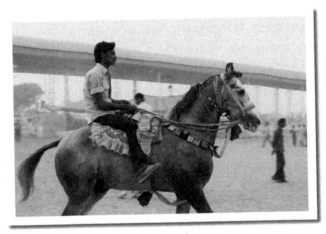

The Revaal

Soon, we are cantering up and down the fields in the dwindling light. My horse has a perfectly relaxed canter. Over and over, I feel waves of relief and pleasure, my confidence restored. The sun is beginning to set, and as I look out across this flat landscape with its occasional acacia, I think of how it is reminiscent of Wisconsin farmland coupled with the exotic elements of Africa, all embraced by the sunset colors of Rajasthan.

MD says the Marwari horse is so fast, "Like a tiger flying after a deer—stretching out like an arrow."

"I'll race you," I suggest, and he's game. We spread out across the field and name the finishing point as a small bush two-thirds of the way down the stretch. Then, we are off. Clearly, MD is going to win, but the thrill of our speed is exhilarating.

When the sun is down, rain begins to lightly fall, dampening our shirts. We walk the horses back to the stable in the mellow, dusky evening light.

At the barn, my horse Arbud is housed next to another young stallion. I walk through a paddock of cattle to get to him, wanting to give both horses a few slices of apple. Arbud seems to enjoy his treat, not realizing, in his equine repose, how well he has treated me and how much gratitude I feel for the hospitality and care of Rohet Garh.

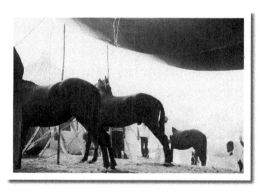

Tent Stable

Jaipur Polo Club

On the way from the Jaipur Airport to the Alsisair Havali, we witness the excitement of the wedding festivities outside the Rambagh Palace. The grand event will take place here later this evening. Reportedly, Nepalese and Indian royalty will be in attendance, along with Hollywood and Bollywood stars, and the writer William Dalrymple, whose book, *Nine Lives: In Search of the Sacred in Modern India*, I am currently reading.

We missed the royal procession that took place earlier that day, but apparently, as the golden vintage chariot moved along, accompanied by decorated elephants, horses, and musicians, lightbulbs flashing at the prince unnerved him so that he was barely able to raise his arm to give the royal salute. The photographers were pushed back to protect him. There is still a crowd of security men and journalists by the front gate—the glorious palace all lit up in the distance.

Ayler appears around ten that night with a beautiful young woman he met in Goa. Kavita Chhabra is of Indian descent, but she was raised in England. She is fluent in Hindi and astonishes the hotel porters as she is still dressed for the beach in short-shorts and a scanty tank top. It is great to see Ayler after this week off on his own, and we quickly begin to catch up on our news.

After an hour of morning yoga on the rooftop terrace, we head to the Gem Palace. The décor here has not been changed for generations—dark wood paneling and glass cabinets. There is a wonderful assortment of affordable jewelry, as well as some astounding pieces. The owner's son, Samir, is a tall, twenty-eight-year-old, in training to take over the business when his father retires. Samir quickly makes friends with Ayler and Kavita, who agree to meet up with him later that night. The owner of the shop graciously invites us up to their rooftop terrace to share some lunch, and it is one of the best meals we have while in India. It makes a difference eating fresh, homemade, vegetarian food.

The following morning we rush to get into the queue for the elephant ride up to the Amber Fort with its impressive golden-yellow walls running for miles across the hills. We stand in line for half-an-hour before we are able to clamber up into the crude metal palanquin set onto the back of our elephant. There are two of us in each basket. But our trek uphill, crushing side-to-side is quite uncomfortable. I continue to smash into Lizbeth the entire way.

After our tour, we head to the Raj Palace Hotel, one of the older and more elegant places in Jaipur. Ayler and Kavita treat us to lunch, and then say that they have a surprise for us. It isn't long before we get it out of them—Samir and his cousin, Sadat, have two horses over at the Jaipur Polo Club, and we are going to be able to ride them that afternoon— *what luck.*

Our amiable driver takes us over to the club where the recently wed prince had his accident five years ago. Everywhere we go we have excellent drivers and guides, but the driving in India is certainly an art form. Most of the roads are difficult, to say the least. Cars are constantly passing trucks in both directions with motorbikes weaving in and out (often with a male driver and wife in back with a child wedged in between). Cows wander about on the roads and passing vehicles head straight at each other only to swerve back into their own proper lanes moments before colliding.

The sky is already darkening as we walk across the massive playing field with Samir and Sadat. We are stopped by an official who says that we are not allowed to walk across the grass. "Rules must be obeyed," he tells us. This is the first time in India that we have heard of any rules. Certainly there are few regulations when it comes to the highway, where artful chaos reigns.

We heed the instructions and walk around the periphery, then find our way back to the encampment of tent stables where the horses are kept. Two horses are brought out, one a black Marwari mare called Chirmi, which means *joyful* in Hindi, and the other, a large grey polo pony, who was originally given the name Maximus, but it was such a difficult word for the grooms to say, they changed it to Mr. John.

I take the Marwari and on mounting notice that the stirrups are very short, and there is no hole-punch available, so there is no way to lengthen the leathers. I make the best of it with my legs cranked up, and begin by walking the mare around the ring where many of the polo ponies are being exercised at a brisk canter. Lizbeth mounts the grey and looks comfortable enough. I try to remember the rules for riding in a ring—isn't it left shoulder to left? Yes, but here in India, where they drive on the opposite side of the road, it is right to right. We quickly get the hang of it.

Chirmi has a nice soft mouth, and she is full of energy. I wonder how her canter will feel, but let her walk out some of her edginess before I move her forward. With the other riders flying by all around me, we get into a nice smooth lope. I keep changing directions, but it's more difficult to get her into a canter using her left lead. The grooms instruct me to put both heels on her side and make a *click-click* sound, and she should respond. Later, when the grooms hop on (one of them in flip-flops), they go flying about the ring.

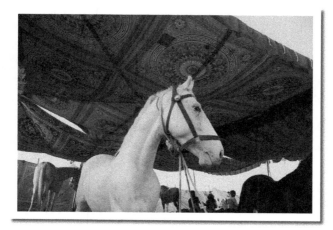

Under Tent

Most of the other horses have been put away by the time we finish up. We all feel exuberant, having had another exciting ride on the last day of our trip. As we leave, the sun is setting on one side of the field, and the moon is rising on the other. Tomorrow, it will be a full moon, another cause for celebration, honoring all the female goddesses in the Hindu religion.

We have had a wonderful trip, but later, heading back to Massachusetts, I think—*some of the best experiences are not always planned and paid for—some of the best rides are waiting for us at home.*

MASSACHUSETTS

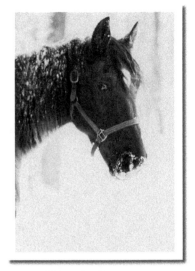

Wintering Barranca

First Snow

Barranca is already growing a thick winter coat so I take him
out slowly through the bare back woods—no more cherry-
colored euonymus, no golden splendor, but the seasonal
change has its own rewards. One can see deeper into the forest.

Wearing my hard hat, my ears are cold, but it is still
enjoyable, enlivening, as the fresh, cold air clears my lungs.
I wrap my long coat around my thighs for warmth. It feels
great having a solid horse between my legs. Big, thick flakes
begin to fall. *First snow descends most silent.*

As we ride the familiar paths, I see a blue rubber glove
by the side of the trail and wonder what it's doing there. Has
it floated to this spot like one of those burst helium balloons?
Or was a hunter wearing it to gut a stag?

I ride down to my mother-in-law's house and wave at her
through the window. She seems happy to see me on my mount

in the falling snow. Soon, we will all be enjoying Christmas Eve together, including Arizona Muse's one-year-old Nikko and hundred-and-one-year-old Emily Rose—much cause for celebration!

Barranca seems glad to be free of the corral. The horses must find this season of hanging around rather dull. Often, they stand at the bottom of the paddock and look in the direction of the lower field. They seem to embody patience.

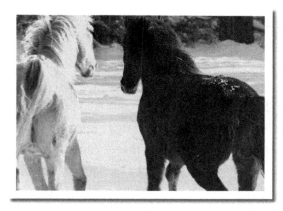

Frisky

Lunar Eclipse

I buy a shooting-star hydrangea for my mother-in-law. While driving it up Rose Hill, the full moon appears through the woods—magnificent. How Em would enjoying seeing that, as she is a lover of all cosmic events, but she is snug in her chair and not going anywhere. When she sees the plant I have brought her, she says simply, "*Star.*"

Today is the winter solstice, the shortest day of the year. The sky is dark by early evening. The lunar eclipse will occur sometime between one and three in the morning. If I were a bit braver and if it wasn't so cold, I would be tempted to take Barranca out for a ride, but it is frigid and windy.

At 1:30 A.M., I put on my heavy coat and double hat and wander down to the corral, giving the horses some treats. I wonder if they are aware that something unusual is going on in the heavens. This kind of eclipse only happens once every four-hundred-and-fifty years. On the other side of the world, all the planets are lined up on either side of the sun forming a chalice. What are we about to receive?

I think about my mother and the freezing distance of space. She is no longer with us but *the earth remembers*—good memories are still warm within me and have not been erased.

Thank you for being honestly passionate, for remaining steadfast, marrying this man, leaping into an unknown world—the cold, often hostile, uninviting North. Thank you for giving birth to the four of us, each a reopening of the caesarian wound. Thank you for being a doting mother when we were babies and could not get too much of your love. Thank you for making a fire each night beneath the painting of the wave-crashing ocean, reading us books, listening to my own early efforts. Thank you for taking us on family vacations, for not smothering us or hovering too closely—giving us freedom, being there when we were hurt— your mad dash to the hospital when I got burned from the exploding Chris Craft. Thank you for the magical Christmases, the stockings and gifts beneath our tinsel-laden tree. Thank you for teaching us manners, no easy task. Thank you for putting up with Oconomowoc so that we could enjoy our extended family. Thank you for not divorcing Popi, for adoring the man he was, even when he was infuriating. Thank you for our wonderful homes, raising us in places of order and beauty. Thank you for remaining so attractive yourself, for greeting our father with a hug and a kiss. Thank you for showing us emotion—letting us know that love is not easy, but that it is always worth it.

Standing out in the freezing cold, Barranca licks my hands, and I rub his neck and forehead. I wait until the moon is completely covered. Light clouds and snowy air bluster by, obscuring clarity so I don't witness the fireball-red surrounding the moon that might be visible elsewhere. The horses seem to prefer standing out in the cold rather than cozying up in their stalls. But I am now ready for a hot, deep tub, with lavender oil brought all the way from Varanasi.

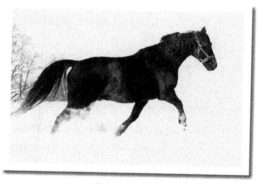

On the Loose

Blizzard Begins

It is truly a joyful Christmas Eve with family and friends gathering down at Em's house. Settling down on the carpet in Em's bedroom, we play the silly game of random present picks and exchanges. Little Nikko passes out gifts to everyone—*what a gem.* Em gets a rather grotesque rhinoceros head made out of plastic, which I found at the dollar store. She examines it with curiosity, perplexed. But then it is Lucy's turn and she takes the rhino away from Em. Perhaps, this hilarity is a bit too much for my mother-in-law, but I know she enjoys the company and the little white lights twinkling on her tree.

Then, on we go to the candlelit dining room with its low ceiling and hearth fire going. The table is decorated with Em's best white linens, china, and silverware, red roses, and holly. We all help ourselves buffet-style to a big, bountiful Christmas meal—squash soup laced with cream and Cointreau for starters, then a perfectly cooked salmon and scalloped potatoes. But in the middle of our intimate dinner, I feel a pang—a poignant sadness—for my mother-in-law. I had a similar feeling when sharing my last meal with my father.

The next day, when everyone leaves for New York, a big winter storm moves into the Berkshires, promising to deliver up to two feet of snow. By mid-afternoon, it is already falling. I am inspired to take one last ride on Barranca through the snowy woods. I bring a kettle of warm water out to the barn to pour over his frozen bit so that it will be more comfortable for him.

It is already getting dark and the blizzard is coming on full force, but I want to ride through this wintry forest one last time. Off we go with wet flakes gathering on my lashes. As we move out at a fast walk, the slanted snow makes it difficult to see—I should have worn ski goggles. But Barranca knows the way and seems to like being out on the trail, even at this hour, even in these conditions. One lone deer springs across the trail—Barranca spots it before I do. I'm glad it survived hunting season, though I wonder how the forest creatures make it through the long, harsh winter and how my big boy will fare. I imagine him drawing into himself and being stalwart, bearing down through the months of ice and snow without complaint. Does he know how much I will miss him?

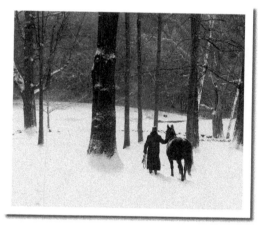

Ready to Leave

ARIZONA

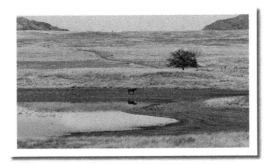

Lone Horse

Epiphany, the Deed is Done

When Mason and I arrive in Patagonia, *Casa Durazno* is freezing cold, no heat. Mason starts up both fires, and we walk around in layers of clothes, retreating to bed with icy noses, shivering. It is almost like sleeping on a grave stone, colder inside than out, colder than Massachusetts.

But today, we have radiant floor heat again, and things are slowly warming up. It is January the sixth, Epiphany, and my friend, Phil Caputo, suggests that this would be a good day to spread my mother's ashes.

I haul Tonka out to the San Rafael for his first ride of the season, tucking the ziplock baggie filled with ashes into my parka pocket. I imagine letting them fly as I ride along. Tonka is ready to go after months of pasture rest, very well-behaved, easy to mount, as the dogs run about in the high grass exploring.

Heading down the dirt road toward Saddle Mountain, where I rode just over a year ago when the Blue Moon rose over the Huachucas, I think about all that happens in the course of a year, and all of the fabulous rides along the way.

More and more, it seems to me that life and death are so intertwined, that all we can do is exist in the moment, pulling that single thread from the warp and the woof of it.

Riding silently, we are alert to the season, the movement, every minute. I'm not sure if I will ever find the last piece of the puzzle or see the whole picture anymore than I do right now— riding across this prairie grassland, solitary yet connected.

Leaving the dirt road, I head out into the field, pulling the baggie from my parka pocket, but the sound of plastic and the ash dust flying immediately spooks my horse. I tense up as he seems ready to bolt or rear. I don't want to be found on the hard desert ground with a broken neck, clutching a ziplock baggie of my mother's ashes, so I ease it back into my parka, and Tonka settles down.

It is a glorious sunny day. There is no one else in sight as I dismount and walk along the fence line, spreading the dusty ashes in the desert grass. It seems a fitting and peaceful place.

There is a tremendous feeling of openness out here in the valley, and I wonder if this simple act will release her. Will she make it to wherever she's going? Is this her last ride or will there be more? What exactly is an epiphany other than the realization that there is something more grand and awesome out there—*Star of Light, Sun of Wonder*. Dust to dust, ashes to ashes, everything living passes. Riding alone, I am content to do so. Who knows where the trail will lead next—*one simply continues.*

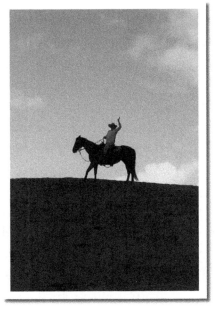

Adios

Cooling the Story Down

After this glorious year in the saddle, riding out on a variety of trails, from the expansive beauty of the Southwest to the lush comforts of the East, I feel that I've attained a kind of midlife bravado with greater self-confidence. Midlife riders have earned this—we have put in time with children, careers, and household chores, but when taking to the trail, we find we are connected to a bigger world.

I now understand more deeply how much the beauty and silence of nature heals me when I ride, lifting me into a meditative state that always puts me in a better mood. Even the same trail, ridden over and over, changes dramatically from one season to the next, and there is always something to witness.

Throughout these pages I have mulled over the past and gained some understanding for the complexity of family. I no longer see my parents in black and white. I no longer feel responsible for their problems. Having forgiven their faults, I've become more aware of my own, and have forgiven myself, also.

Over the past year, I have learned to call it quits when a ride seemed too dangerous. Perhaps I've moved on from being an acquiescent child to becoming a more responsible adult, a little less naïve about the potential mishaps that can occur while riding. Certainly anything can happen on a horse, and the unexpected is to *be* expected.

There is no counting on the timing of things. You never know when a beloved family member will pass or when a butterfly might appear. Emily Rose, my dear mother-in-law, made it to her one-hundred-and-second birthday, then died four hours later. She taught me so much about appreciating life—raising her hands in delight before a cloud formation, a tree laden with apples, a view, a taste, a bouquet of flowers— how every gesture and arrangement should acknowledge transience and evoke the beautiful.

Recently, I returned to the place where I spread my mother's ashes and had a good cry. Finally, I felt connected to my own sadness, capable of mourning her. I should have had more compassion for her while she was still alive. I should have reached out and told her that I understood her loneliness.

Often, I have wanted to pick up the phone and give her a call—*Mom, this is your daughter, Laura.* I feel that if she could answer, she would wish me well, that she would want happiness for me just as she had wanted it for herself.

Witnessing life as it passes makes me want to enter the moment, and what better way to do that than riding out into nature, out into the elements, breathing in the forest air— riding *all out* with gratitude and joy, every day that we are able.

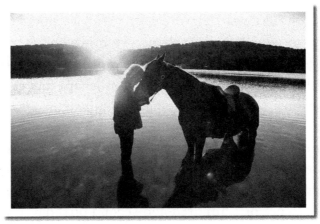

End of Day

ACKNOWLEDGMENTS

My closest cousin, Helen Chester, was my most frequent riding partner during the year of this account. Her relaxed and easygoing manner made for many leisurely, enjoyable rides. My thanks also go out to the many other friends who joined me on the trail—Phil Caputo, Leslie Ware, Elizabeth Beautyman, Lizbeth Marano, Ayler Young, Betsy Spears, Avia Rose Stanton, Arizona Muse, Donna DeMari, Kacy Brehm and Keith Warner, Melinda South, Betsy Pettit, Erma Duran, Teri Arnold Shannon and Rosemary Kovatch, Anita Cloveski-Wharton, Peter Phinney, Cia and Abigail McKoy, Kevin Crowe, and Daphne Chester. You were all great riding companions! My special gratitude goes to Jill Johnson and Summer Brenner for their enduring friendship and careful readings of the manuscript in progress. I also want to thank Martha Cook, and Caroline Robbins of Trafalgar Square Books, as well as senior editor Rebecca Didier for her insightful direction, which helped me shape this book in its final stages. Loving gratitude goes to Wanda White, my mother's devoted caregiver, and to my darling sister Cia who managed our mother's medical and personal issues during the last years of her life. Finally, I know this book wouldn't be what it is without the wonderful, revealing photographs of my dear friend Donna DeMari and my husband Mason Rose.

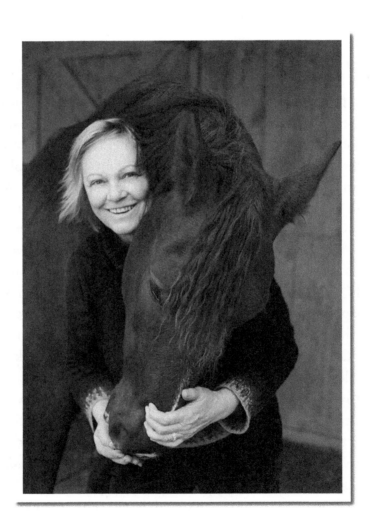

ABOUT THE AUTHOR

Laura Chester has published many volumes of poetry, prose and non-fiction. Most recently, a book of short stories, *Rancho Weirdo*, became available from Bootstrap Press. Editor of six anthologies, her latest collections are *Eros & Equus, a passion for the horse*, and *Heartbeat for Horses*, both from Willow Creek Press, including extensive photographs by Donna DeMari. Indiana University Press published the non-fiction book, *Holy Personal, looking for small private places of worship*, while Station Hill Press released an updated version of *Lupus Novice, toward self-healing*, an account of Chester's personal struggle and breakthrough with the auto-immune disease SLE. Other recent books include *The Stone Baby*, and *Bitches Ride Alone*, Black Sparrow Press; *The Story of the Lake*, Faber & Faber; *Kingdom Come*, Creative Arts; and *Sparks*, The Figures. Having grown up in Milwaukee and Oconomowoc, Wisconsin, Chester now lives in Patagonia, Arizona and the Berkshires of Massachusetts.